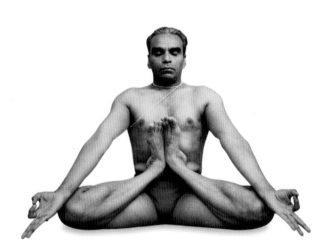

Iyengar
Yoga
for beginners

Iyengar Yoga

for beginners

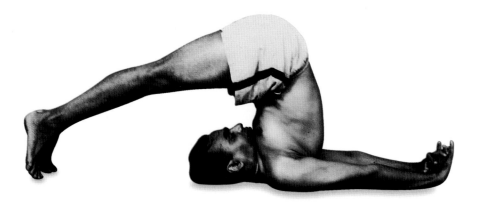

An introduction to the classic poses

B.K.S. IYENGAR

DORLING KINDERSLEY
LONDON, NEW YORK, MELBOURNE
MUNICH and DELHI

PROJECT EDITOR: Ranjana Sengupta
PROJECT DESIGNER: Aparna Sharma
EDITORS: Dipali Singh, Sheema Mookherjee, Larissa Sayers
DESIGNERS: Ankita Saha, Nikki Duggal
DTP DESIGNER: Sunil Sharma, Pankaj Sharma, Harish Aggarwal
MANAGING EDITOR: Prita Maitra
MANAGING EDITOR (UK): Penny Warren
MANAGING ART EDITOR: Shuka Jain
MANAGING ART EDITOR (UK): Marianne Markham

B. K. S. Iyengar would like to thank: Dr Geeta S. Iyengar for her contribution to editing the script and assisting with the photography; Parth Amin; for his ideas, and perseverance in completing the book; Prof. R. N. Kulhali, for drafting and compiling the Yoga text; Zarina Kolah, Yoga Consultant, for her help in compiling the text and liaising with the DK editorial team; Harminder Singh for the photography; and models Roshen Amin, Leslie Peters, Ali Dashti, and Jawahar Bangera.

First published in Great Britain in 2006

by Dorling Kindersley Limited,
80 Strand, London WC2R ORL
Penguin Group (UK)

6 8 10 9 7

Material in this publication was previously published by Dorling Kindersley in *Yoga: the Path to Holistic Health* by B.K.S. Iyengar

A CIP catalogue record for this book is available from the British Library.

ISBN-13: 978-1-40531-738-2

Reproduced by Colourscan, Singapore
Printed in Singapore by Star Standard

Discover more at
www.dk.com

Contents

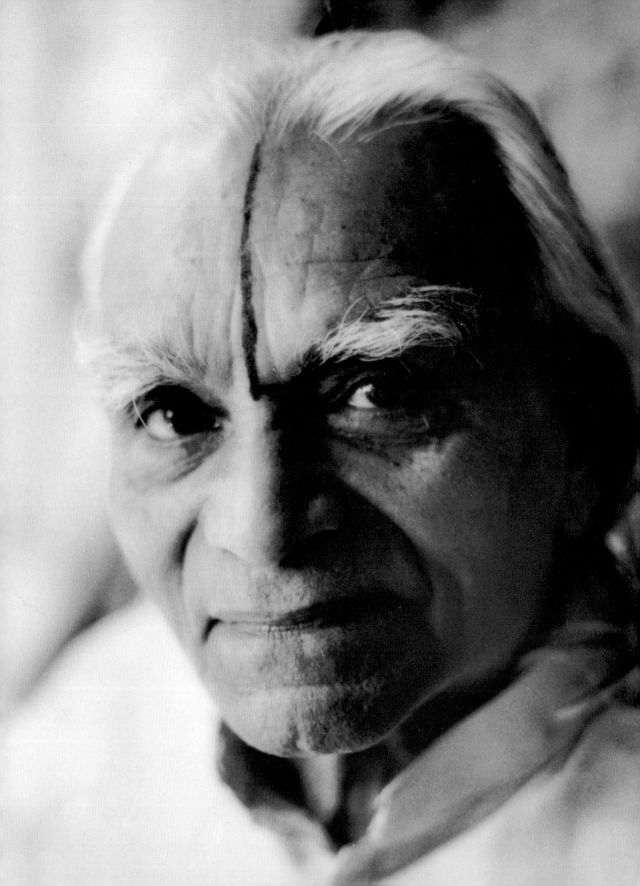

FOREWORD

by Yogacharya B.K.S. Iyengar

Yoga is for everyone. You need not be an expert or at the peak of physical fitness to practise the asanas described in this book. The strain of modern life can lead to physical pain and illness, as we neglect our bodies in the race for material success. The stress of modern life can also lead to mental suffering: feelings of inadequacy, isolation, or powerlessness. Yoga helps to integrate the mental and the physical plane, bringing about a sense of inner and outer balance, or what I term *alignment*. True alignment means that the inner mind reaches every cell and fibre of the body.

During my 70 years of teaching and practising, I have observed that some students pay attention only to the physical aspect of yoga. Their practice is like a fast-flowing stream, tumbling and falling, which lacks depth and direction. By attending to the mental and spiritual side, a sincere student of yoga becomes like a smoothly flowing river which helps to irrigate and fertilize the land around it. Just as one cannot dip into the same river twice, so each and every asana refreshes your life force with new energy.

My effort in this book has been to focus on techniques, so that even the beginner will have a thorough understanding of how to practise asanas in order to obtain the maximum benefit. By using a few simple props, students with different capabilities can gradually build up strength, confidence, and flexibility without the threat of strain or injury. The yoga techniques described and illustrated in this book can also help those with specific ailments. Regular practice builds up the body's inner strength and natural resistance, helps to alleviate pain, and tackles the root, rather than the symptoms, of the problem. Across the world, there is now a growing awareness that alternative therapies are more conducive to health than conventional ones. It is my hope that this book will help all those who want to change their lives through yoga. May yoga's blessing be on all of you.

CHAPTER 1

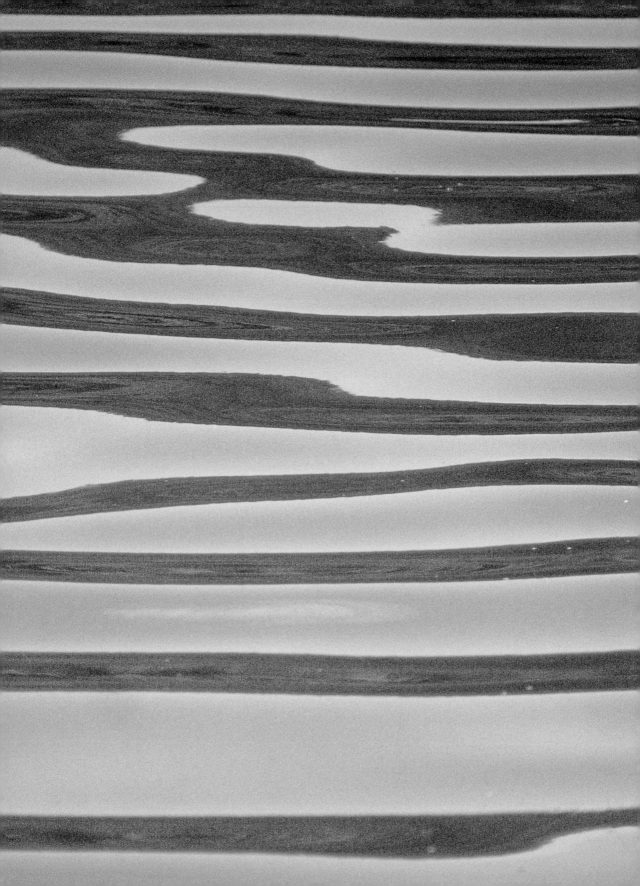

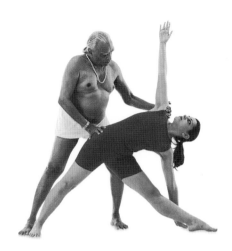

"Yoga is a light which, once lit, will never dim. The better your practice, the brighter the flame."

Yoga for You

The primary aim of yoga is to restore the mind to simplicity and peace, to free it from confusion and distress. This sense of calm comes from the practice of yogic asanas and pranayama. Unlike other forms of exercise which strain muscles and bones, yoga gently rejuvenates the body. By restoring the body, yoga frees the mind from the negative feelings caused by the fast pace of modern life. The practice of yoga fills up the reservoirs of hope and optimism within you. It helps you to overcome all obstacles on the path to perfect health and spiritual contentment. It is a rebirth.

Aims of Yoga

The practice of yoga aims at overcoming the limitations of the body.
Yoga teaches us that the goal of every individual's life is to take the inner journey
to the soul. Yoga offers both the goal and the means to reach it.

When there is perfect harmony between body and mind, we achieve self-realization. Yoga teaches us that obstacles in the path of our self-realization indicate themselves in physical or mental indisposition. When our physical state is not perfect, this causes an imbalance in our mental state, which is known in Sanskrit as *chittavritti*. The practice of yoga helps us to overcome that imbalance. Yogic asanas, or poses, can cure *vyadhi* or physical ailments, and redress *angamejayatva* or unsteadiness in the body. *Shvasa-prashvasa*, which translates as "uneven respiration" – an indication of stress – is alleviated by the practice of yoga. Asanas tone the whole body. They strengthen bones and muscles, correct posture, improve breathing, and increase energy. This physical well-being has a strengthening and calming impact on the mind.

ASANAS AND PRANAYAMA

Practising asanas cleanses the body. Just as a goldsmith heats gold in fire to burn out its impurities, similarly, asanas, by increasing the circulation of fresh blood through the body, purge it of the diseases and toxins which are the consequences of an irregular lifestyle, unhealthy habits, and poor posture. Regular practice of the stretches, twists, bends, and inversions – the basic movements of asanas – restores strength and stamina to the body. Asanas, together with pranayama, or the control of breath, rectify physical, physiological, and psychological disorders. They have a positive impact on the effects of stress and disease. Among the many ailments that benefit from the practice of asanas are osteoarthritis, high and low blood pressure, diabetes, asthma, and anorexia.

HARMONY BETWEEN BODY AND SOUL
This 10th-century figure, the Yoga Narayan,
from Khajuraho, India, depicts the god Vishnu
in a state of yogic calm

MIND AND BODY

The body and the mind are in a state of constant interaction. Yogic science does not demarcate where the body ends and the mind begins, but approaches both as a single, integrated entity. The turmoil of daily life brings stress to the body and the mind. This creates anxiety, depression, restlessness, and rage. Yoga asanas, while appearing to deal with the physical body alone, actually influence the chemical balance of the brain, which in turn improves one's mental state of being.

The obstacles to this perfect balance were outlined by the sage, Patanjali, some 2,000 years ago in the *Yoga Sutras*. Historians disagree on the exact dates, but it is known that the *sutras*, or aphorisms on the philosophy and practice of yoga, were compiled sometime between 300 BC and AD 300, and the entire corpus was called the *Patanjala Yoga Darshana*. In the final chapter of the *Yoga Sutras*, the *Samadhi Pada*, Patanjali discusses the disorders that are the root cause of suffering. According to the sage, *vyadhi* or physical ailments, create emotional upheaval. The task of yoga is to tackle both.

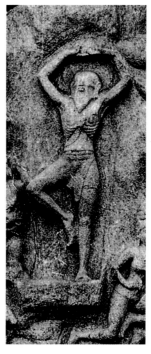
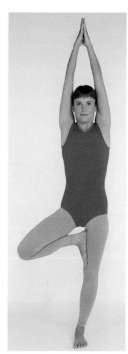

TIMELESS TRADITION
The 4th-century figure from Mahabalipuram, India (left), and this modern woman show that certain classic movements are eternal

> ## "*After a session of yoga, the mind becomes tranquil and passive.*"

The alleviation of pain is, even today, one of the main reasons for the journey into yoga for most people. Yoga asanas work specific parts of the body to soothe and relax the mind as well. Inverted asanas, for instance, simultaneously calm and stimulate the brain. These asanas activate glands and vital organs by supplying fresh blood to the brain, making it alert but relaxed.

Yoga possesses the unique ability to calm the nerves. The nerves function as the medium between the physiological body and the psychological body (*see page 42*). Practising yoga has the holistic impact of relaxing the body and calming the mind.

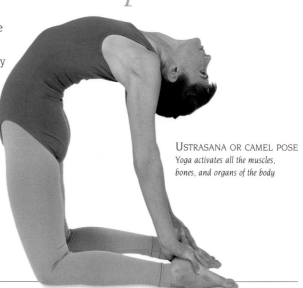

USTRASANA OR CAMEL POSE
Yoga activates all the muscles, bones, and organs of the body

STAGES OF YOGA

The primary aim of yoga is to restore the mind to simplicity, peace, and poise, to free it from confusion and distress. This simplicity, this sense of order and calm, comes from the practice of asanas and pranayama. Yoga asanas integrate the body, the mind, the intelligence and, finally, the self, in four stages. The first stage, *arambhavastha*, is one in which we practise at the level of the physical body. The second stage is *ghatavastha*, when the mind learns to move in unison with the body. The third level, *parichayavastha*, occurs when the intelligence and the body become one. The final stage is *nishpattyavastha*, the state of perfection (*see page 42*).

Spiritual awareness flows into the student of yoga through these stages. *Duhkha*, which is misery or pain, vanishes, and the art of living in simplicity and peace is realized.

YOGA FILLS THE SPIRITUAL VOID

The world today is overwhelmingly materialistic, and this has created a great spiritual void in our lives. Our lifestyles are unduly complex and we become stressed primarily as a result of our own actions. Our existence feels barren and devoid of meaning. There is a lack of spiritual dimension to our lives and in our relationships. This has led many reflective people to realize that solace and inspiration, peace and happiness, cannot come from the external environment but must come from within.

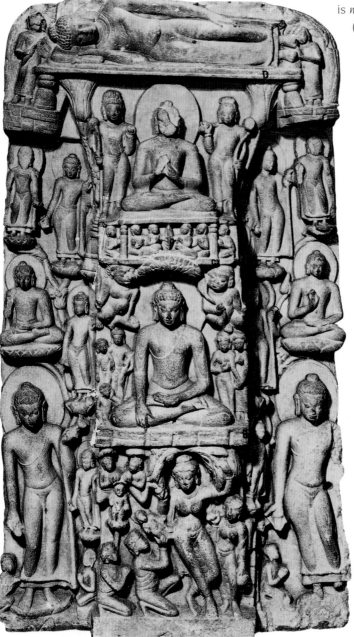

THE FOUR STAGES OF THE BUDDHA'S JOURNEY TO SELF-REALIZATION
This 5th-century frieze from Sarnath, India, shows the four defining events of the Buddha's life. (From the bottom) Buddha's birth from his mother's hip; attaining enlightenment in Bodhgaya; preaching to his disciples; the ascent to the celestial realms

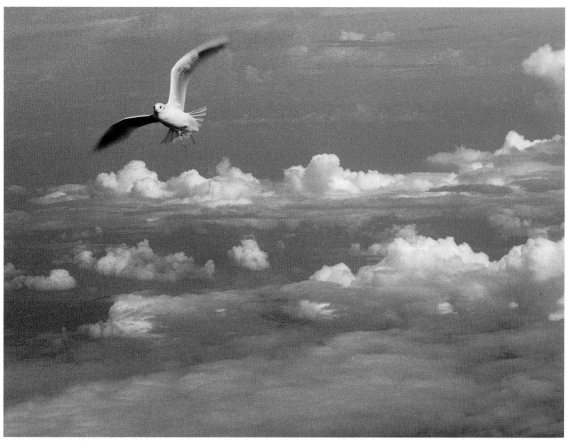

YOGA LIBERATES YOU
When you practise yoga, your mind becomes unfettered and free

THE FREEDOM OF YOGA

The impact of yoga is never purely physical. Asanas, if correctly practised, bridge the divide between the physical and the mental spheres. Yoga stems the feelings of pain, fatigue, doubt, confusion, indifference, laziness, self-delusion, and despair that assail us from time to time. The yogic mind simply refuses to accept such negative emotions and seeks to overcome these turbulent currents on the voyage to the total liberation of the self. Once we become sincere practitioners of yoga, we cease to be tormented by these unhappy and discouraging states of mind.

Yoga illuminates your life. If you practise sincerely, with seriousness and honesty, its light will spread to all aspects of your life. Regular practice will bring you to look at yourself and your goals in a new light. It will help remove the obstacles to good health and stable emotions. In this way, yoga will help you to achieve emancipation and self-realization, which is the ultimate goal of every person's life.

UNWAVERING FLAME
Yoga illuminates your life, helping you to see yourself in a new light

Meaning of Yoga

Yoga is an ancient art based on an extremely subtle science, that of the body, mind, and soul. The prolonged practice of yoga will, in time, lead the student to a sense of peace and a feeling of being at one with his or her environment.

Most people know that the practice of yoga makes the body strong and flexible. It is also well known that yoga improves the functioning of the respiratory, circulatory, digestive, and hormonal systems. Yoga also brings emotional stability and clarity of mind, but that is only the beginning of the journey to *samadhi*, or self-realization, which is the ultimate aim of yoga.

The ancient sages, who meditated on the human condition 2,000 years ago, outlined four ways to self-realization: *jnana marg*, or the path to knowledge, when the seeker learns to discriminate between the real and the unreal; *karma marg*, the path of selfless service without thought of reward; *bhakti marg*, the path of love and devotion; and finally, *yoga marg*, the path by which the mind and its actions are brought under control. All these paths lead to the same goal: *samadhi*.

The word "yoga" is derived from the Sanskrit root *yuj* which means "to join" or "to yoke"; the related meaning is "to focus attention on" or "to use". In philosophical terms, the union of the individual self, *jivatma*, with the universal self, *paramatma*, is yoga. The union results in a pure and perfect state of consciousness in which the feeling of "I" simply does not exist. Prior to this union is the union of the body with the mind, and the mind with the self. Yoga is thus a dynamic, internal experience which integrates the body, the senses, the mind, and the intelligence, with the self.

The sage Patanjali was a master of yoga and a fully evolved soul. But this great thinker had the ability to empathize with the joys and sorrows of ordinary people. His reflections and those of other ancient sages on the ways through which every person could realize his full potential were outlined in the 196 *Yoga Sutras*.

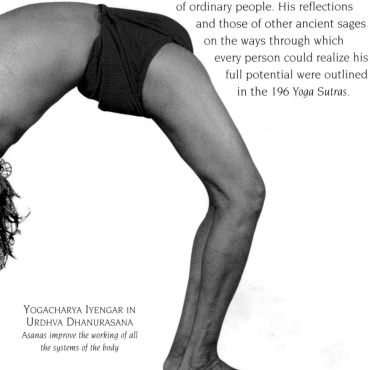

YOGACHARYA IYENGAR IN
URDHVA DHANURASANA
*Asanas improve the working of all
the systems of the body*

WHERE YOGA CAN TAKE YOU

According to Patanjali, the aim of yoga is to calm the chaos of conflicting impulses and thoughts. The mind, which is responsible for our thoughts and impulses, is naturally inclined to *asmita* or egoism. From this spring the prejudice and biases which lead to pain and distress in our daily lives. Yogic science centres the intelligence in two areas: the heart and the head. The intelligence of the heart, sometimes also called the "root mind", is the actual agent of *ahankara* or false pride, which disturbs the intelligence of the head, causing fluctuations in the body and mind.

Patanjali describes these afflictions as: *vyadhi* or physical ailments, *styana* or the reluctance to work, *samshaya* or doubt, *pramada* or indifference, *alasya* or laziness, *avirati* or the desire for sensual satisfaction, *bharanti darshana* or false knowledge, *alabdha bhumikatva* or indisposition, *angamejayatva* or unsteadiness in the body, and, lastly, *shvasa-prashvasa* or unsteady respiration. Only yoga eradicates these afflictions, and disciplines the mind, emotions, intellect, and reason.

ASTANGA YOGA

Yoga is also known as Astanga yoga. A*stanga* means "8 limbs" or "steps" (*see page* 29) and is divided into 3 disciplines. The discipline, *bahiranga-sadhana*, comprises ethical practices in the form of *yama*, or general ethical principles, *niyama*, or self-restraint, and physical practices in the form of asanas as well as pranayama.

The second discipline, *antaranga-sadhana*, is emotional or mental discipline brought to maturity by pranayama and *pratyahara*, or mental detachment. Lastly, *antaratma-sadhana* is the successful quest of the soul through *dharana*, *dhyana*, and *samadhi* (*see page 29*).

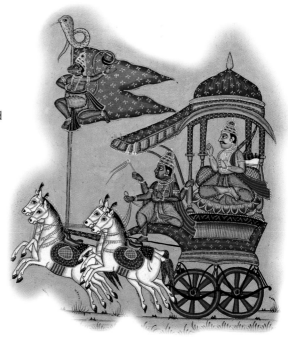

KRISHNA DRIVING THE CHARIOT OF THE WARRIOR, ARJUN
Their discourses are narrated in the Bhagvad Gita, *the main source of yogic philosophy*

In this spiritual quest, it is important to remember the role of the body. The *Kathopanishad*, an ancient text compiled between 300–400 BC, compares the body to a chariot, the senses to the horses, and the mind to the reins. The intellect is the charioteer and the soul is the master of the chariot. If anything were to go wrong with the chariot, the horses, the reins, or the charioteer, the chariot and the charioteer would come to grief, and so would the master of the chariot.

But, writes Patanjali in *Yoga Sutra* 11.28, "The practice of yoga destroys the impurities of the body and mind, after which maturity in intelligence and wisdom radiate from the core of the being to function in unison with the body, senses, mind, intelligence, and the consciousness."

"The aim of yoga is to calm the chaos of conflicting impulses."

The Way to Health

Good health results from perfect communication between each part of the body and mind; when each cell communes with every other. Although yoga is essentially a spiritual science, it leads to a sense of physical and emotional well-being.

Health is not just freedom from disease. For good health, the joints, tissues, muscles, cells, nerves, glands, and each system of the body must all be in a state of perfect balance and harmony. Health is the perfect equilibrium of the body and mind, intellect, and soul.

Health is like the flowing water of a river, always fresh and pure, in a constant state of flux. Humans are a combination of the senses of perception, the organs of action, the mind, the intelligence, the inner consciousness, and the conscience. Each of these is worked on by the practice of yoga.

Yoga asanas help to ensure an even distribution of bio-energy, or life-force, which brings the mind to a state of calm. A practitioner of yoga faces life not as a victim, but as a master, in control of his or her life situations, circumstances, and environment.

Asanas balance the respiratory, circulatory, nervous, hormonal, digestive, excretory, and reproductive systems perfectly. The equilibrium in the body then brings mental peace and enhances intellectual clarity.

GOOD HEALTH
A healthy body is like the flowing water of a river - always fresh and pure

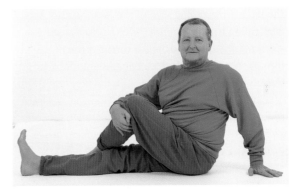

YOGA IS FOR EVERYONE
There are asanas to suit every constitution, irrespective of age or physical condition

HARMONY OF BODY AND MIND

Asanas cater to the needs of each individual according to his or her specific constitution and physical condition. They involve vertical, horizontal, and cyclical movements, which provide energy to the system by directing the blood supply to the areas of the body which need it most. In yoga, each cell is observed, attended to, and provided with a fresh supply of blood, allowing it to function smoothly.

The mind is naturally active and dynamic, while the soul is luminous. However, unhealthy bodies tend to house inert, dull, and sluggish minds. It is the practice of yoga which removes this sluggishness from the body and brings it to the level of the active mind. Ultimately, both the body and mind rise to the level of the illuminated self.

The practice of yoga stimulates and changes emotional attitudes, converting apprehensiveness into courage, indecision and poor judgement into positive decision-making skills, and emotional instability into confidence and mental equilibrium.

Benefits of Poses

Asanas are based on the three basic human postures of standing, sitting, or lying down. But they are not a series of movements to be followed mechanically. They have a logic which must be internalized if the pose is to be practised correctly.

The Sanskrit term, *asana*, is sometimes translated as "pose" and sometimes as "posture". Neither translation is wholly accurate, as they do not convey the element of thought or consciousness that must inform each movement of the asana. The final pose of an asana is achieved when all the parts of the body are positioned correctly, with full awareness and intelligence.

To achieve this, you must think through the structure of the asana. Realize the fundamental points by imagining how you will adjust and arrange each part of your anatomical body, especially the limbs, in the given movements.

Then, mould the body to fit the structure of the asana, making sure that the balance between both sides of the body is perfect, until there is no undue stress on any one organ, muscle, bone, or joint.

IMPORTANCE OF PRACTISING ASANAS

The practice of asanas has a beneficial impact on the whole body. Asanas not only tone the muscles, tissues, ligaments, joints, and nerves, but also maintain the smooth functioning and health of all the body's systems. They relax the body and mind, allowing both to recover from fatigue or weakness, and the stress of daily life. Asanas also boost metabolism, lymphatic circulation, and hormonal secretions, and bring about a chemical balance in the body.

It is important to keep practising until you are absolutely comfortable in the final pose. It is only then that you experience the full benefits of the asana. The sage Patanjali observes in *Yoga Sutra* 11.47, "Perfection in an asana is achieved when the effort to perform it becomes effortless, and the infinite being within is reached."

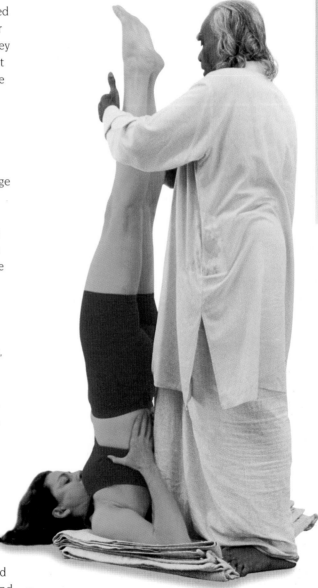

PERFECT BALANCE
Yogacharya Iyengar supports a student in Salamba Sarvangasana

Yoga & Fitness

Most types of exercise are competitive. Yoga, although non-competitive, is nevertheless challenging. The challenge is to one's own will power. It is a competition between one's self and one's body.

Exercise usually involves quick and forceful body movements. It has repeated actions which often lead to exertion, tension, and fatigue. Yoga asanas, on the other hand, involve movements which bring stability to the body, the senses, the mind, the intellect, the consciousness, and finally, to the conscience. The very essence of an asana is steady movement, a process that does not simply end, but finds fulfilment in tranquillity.

Most diseases are caused by the fluctuations in the brain and in the behavioural pattern of the body. In yogic practice, the brain is quietened, the senses are stilled, and perceptions are altered, all generating a calm feeling of detachment. With practice, the student of yoga learns to treat the brain as an object and the body as a subject. Energy is diffused from the brain to the other parts of the body. The brain and body then work together and

energy is evenly balanced between the two. Yoga is thus termed *sarvaanga sadhana* or "holistic practice". No other form of exercise so completely involves the mind and self with the body, resulting in all-round development and harmony. Other forms of exercise address only particular parts of the body. Such forms are termed *angabhaga sadhana* or "physical exercise".

STIMULATIVE EXERCISE

Yoga asanas are stimulative exercises, while other endurance exercises are irritative. For instance, medical experts claim that jogging stimulates the heart. In fact, though the heartbeat of the jogger increases, the heart is not stimulated in the yogic sense of being energized and invigorated. In yoga, back bends, for example, are more physically demanding than jogging, but the heart beats at a steady, rhythmic pace.

Asanas do not lead to breathlessness. When practising yoga, strength and power play separate roles to achieve a perfect balance in every part of the body, as well as the mind. After such stimulating exercise, a sense of rejuvenation and a fresh surge of energy follow.

Exercise can also be exhausting. Many forms of exercise require physical strength and endurance and can lead to a feeling of fatigue after 10-15 minutes of practice. Many such exercises improve energy levels by boosting nerve function, but ultimately, this exhausts the cellular reserves and the endocrine glands. Cellular toxins increase, and though circulation is enhanced, it is at the cost of irritating the other body systems and increasing the pulse rate and blood pressure. Ultimately, the heart is taxed and overworked.

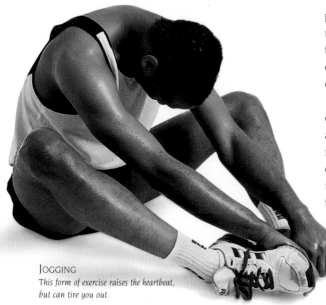

JOGGING
This form of exercise raises the heartbeat, but can tire you out

An athlete's strong lung capacity is achieved by hard and forceful usage, which is not conducive to preserving the health of the lungs. Furthermore, ordinary physical exercise, such as in jogging, tennis, or football, lends itself to repetitive injuries of the bones, joints, and ligaments.

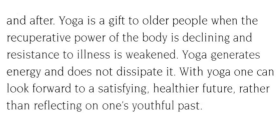

STRENGTHENING IMMUNITIES
Children benefit from yoga as much as adults do

Such forms of exercise work with – and for – the skeletal and muscular systems. They cannot penetrate beyond these limits. But asanas penetrate each layer of the body and, ultimately, the consciousness itself. Only in yoga can you keep both the body and the mind relaxed, even as you stretch, extend, rotate, and flex your body.

Yoga, unlike other forms of exercise, keeps the nervous system elastic and capable of bearing stress. Although all forms of exercise bring about a feeling of well-being, they also stress the body. Yoga refreshes the body, while other systems exhaust it. Yoga involves the equal exertion of all parts of the body and does not overstrain any one part.

In other forms of exercise, the movements are restricted to a part or parts. They are reflex actions, which do not involve the intelligence in their execution. There is little space for precision and perfection, without extra expenditure of energy.

YOGA CAN BE PRACTISED AT ANY AGE

With advancing age, physically vigorous exercises cannot be performed easily because of stiffening joints and muscles that have lost tone. Isometric exercises, for example, cannot be practised with increasing age, as they lead to sprained muscles, painful joints, strained body systems, and the degeneration of organs. The great advantage of yoga is that it can be practised by anyone, irrespective of age, sex, and physical condition.

In fact, yoga is particularly beneficial in middle age

and after. Yoga is a gift to older people when the recuperative power of the body is declining and resistance to illness is weakened. Yoga generates energy and does not dissipate it. With yoga one can look forward to a satisfying, healthier future, rather than reflecting on one's youthful past.

Unlike other exercises, yoga results in the concentration of immunity cells in areas affected by disease, and thus improves immunity. That is why the ancient sages called yoga a therapeutic as well as a preventive science.

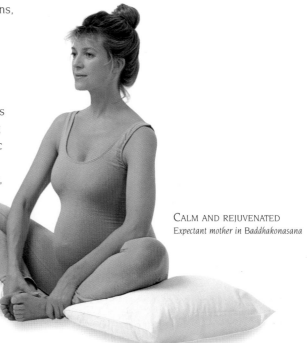

CALM AND REJUVENATED
Expectant mother in Baddhakonasana

Yoga & Stress

Yoga minimizes the impact of stress on the individual. Yogic science believes that the regular practice of asanas and pranayama strengthens the nervous system and helps people face stressful situations positively.

We have all experienced the way unrelieved tension results in both mental disorders and physical ill-health. This is not a modern phenomenon. In the centuries-old *Yoga Sutras*, the sage Patanjali attributed the causes of mental affliction to the ego, spiritual ignorance, desire, hatred of others, and attachment to life. He called these *kleshas* or "sorrows".

ORIGINS OF STRESS

Through advances in science and technology, modern civilization has been able to conquer ignorance in many fields, but its pride in

grasp at in their desperate search for consolation. But while these measures may provide temporary distraction or oblivion, the root cause of unhappiness – stress – remains unresolved.

Yoga is not a miracle cure that can free a person from all stress, but it can help to minimize it. The worries of modern life deplete our reserves of bio-energy, because we draw on our vital energy from the storehouse – the nerve cells. This can, ultimately, exhaust our energy reserves and lead to the collapse of mental and physical equilibrium.

Yogic science believes that the nerves control the unconscious mind, and that when the nervous

> "*Regular practice of yoga can help you face the turmoil of life with steadiness and stability.*"

technological achievement is excessive and misplaced. It has triggered widespread feelings of competitiveness and envy. Financial tensions, emotional upheavals, environmental pollution and, above all, a sense of being overtaken by the speed of events, have all increased the stress of daily life.

All these factors strain the body, causing nervous tension, and adversely affecting the mind. This is when feelings of isolation and loneliness take over.

To deal with this, people turn to artificial solutions to cope with the pressures of daily life. Substance abuse, eating disorders, and destructive relationships are some of the substitutes people

system is strong, a person faces stressful situations more positively. Asanas improve blood flow to all the cells of the body, revitalizing the nerve cells. This flow strengthens the nervous system and its capacity for enduring stress.

RELIEVING STRESS

The diaphragm, according to yogic science, is the seat of the intelligence of the heart and the window to the soul. During stressful situations, however, when you inhale and exhale, the diaphragm becomes too taut to alter its shape. Yogic exercises address this problem by developing elasticity in the diaphragm, so that, when stretched, it can handle any amount of stress, whether intellectual, emotional, or physical.

The practice of asanas and pranayama helps to integrate the body, breath, mind, and intellect. Slow, effortless exhalation during practice of an asana brings serenity to the body cells, relaxes the facial muscles, and releases all tension from the organs of perception: the eyes, ears, nose, tongue, and skin.

When this happens, the brain, which is in constant communication with the organs of action, becomes *shunya*, or void, and all thoughts are stilled. Then, invading fears and anxieties cannot penetrate to the brain. When you develop this ability, you perform your daily activities with efficiency and economy. You do not dissipate your valuable bio-energy. You enter the state of true clarity of intellect. Your mind is free of stress and is filled with calm and tranquillity.

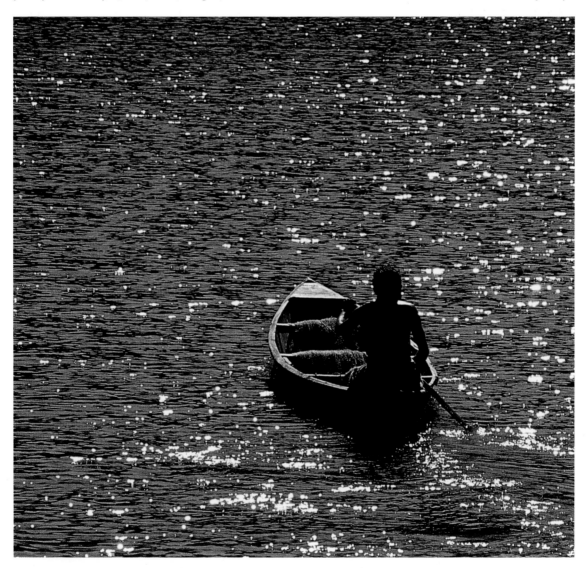

A VIEW OF THE SOUL
Yoga can minimize the worries of modern life

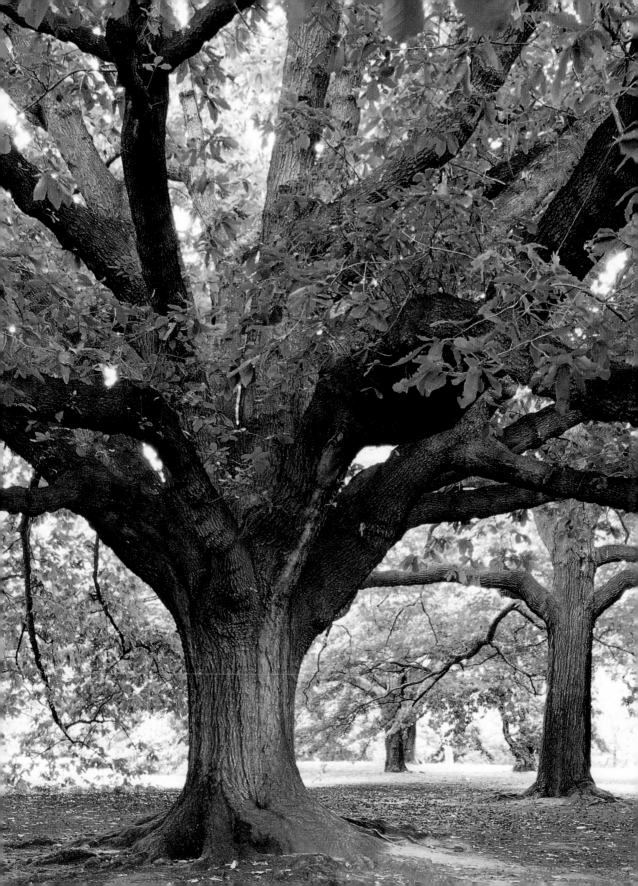

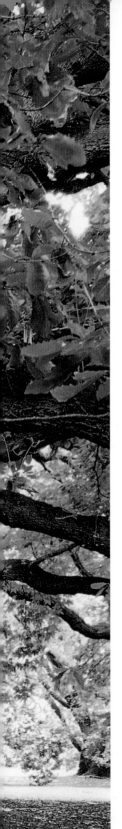

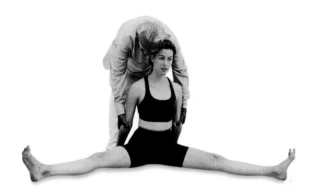

CHAPTER 2

"Yoga is the union of the individual self with the universal self."

Philosophy of Yoga

Yoga is a fine art and seeks to express the artist's abilities to the fullest possible extent. While most artists need an instrument, such as a paintbrush or a violin, to express their art, the only instruments a yogi needs are his body and his mind. The ancient sages compared yoga to a fruit tree. From a single seed grow the roots, trunk, branches, and leaves. The leaves bring life-giving energy to the entire tree, which then blossoms into flowers and sweet, luscious fruit. Just as the fruit is the natural culmination of the tree, yoga, too, transforms darkness into light, ignorance into knowledge, knowledge into wisdom, and wisdom into unalloyed peace and spiritual bliss.

Philosophy of Asanas

Asanas, one of yoga's most significant "tools", help the sincere student develop physically and spiritually. The ancient sages believed that if you put your whole heart into your practice, you become a master of your circumstances and time.

Asanas are one of the major "tools" of yoga. Their benefits range from the physical level to the spiritual. That is why yoga is called *sarvaanga sadhana*, or holistic practice. "Asana" is the positioning of the body in various postures, with the total involvement of the mind and self, in order to establish communication between our external and internal selves.

Yogic philosophy looks at the body as being made up of three layers and five sheaths. The three layers are: the causal body, or *karana sharira*, the subtle body, or *suksma sharira*, and the gross body, or *karya sharira*. Every individual functions in mind, matter, energy, and pure consciousness through five sheaths. These are: the anatomical sheath, or *annamaya kosha*, which is dealt with by asanas; the life-force sheath or *pranamaya kosha*, which is treated by pranayama; the psychological sheath, or *manomaya kosha*, is worked on by meditation; and the intellectual sheath, or *vijnamaya kosha*, is transformed by studying the scriptures with sincerity and discrimination. Once these goals are addressed, you reach the *anandamaya kosha*, or the sheath of bliss.

Yoga integrates the three layers of the body with the five sheaths, enabling the individual to develop as a total being. The separation between the body and the mind, and the mind and the soul, then vanishes, as all planes fuse into one. In this way, asanas help to transform an individual by bringing him or her away from the awareness of the body toward the consciousness of the soul.

THE JOURNEY OF YOGA

The *Hathayoga Pradipika* is a practical treatise on yoga, thought to have been compiled in the 15th century. The author, the sage Svatmarama, gives practical guidelines to beginners on the journey they must make from the culture of the body toward the vision of the soul. Unlike Patanjali, who discusses the sighting of the soul through the restraint of consciousness or *chitta*, Svatmarama begins his treatise with the restraint of energy, or *prana*. Sighting the soul through the restraint of energy is called Hatha yoga, whereas sighting the soul through the restraint of consciousness is known as Raja yoga.

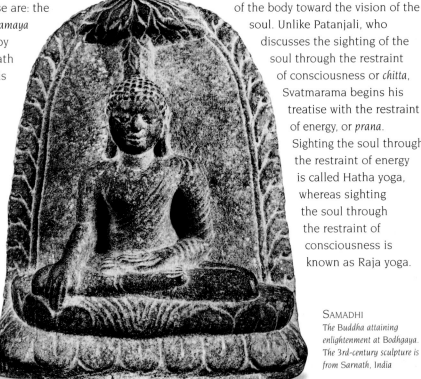

SAMADHI
The Buddha attaining enlightenment at Bodhgaya. The 3rd-century sculpture is from Sarnath, India

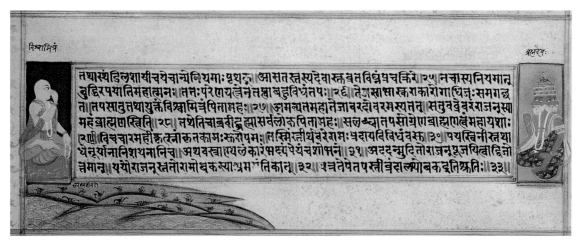

A FOLIO FROM THE ANCIENT INDIAN EPIC, THE MAHABHARATA.
The essentials of yoga philosophy are found in the Bhagvad Gita, which forms a part of the epic

In *Hathayoga Pradipika* 4.29, the author stresses the importance of the breath by saying that if the mind is the king of the senses, the master of the mind is breath. If breath is made to move rhythmically, with a controlled, sustained sound, the mind becomes calm. In that calmness, the king of the mind (the soul) becomes the supreme commander of the senses, mind, breath, as well as consciousness. When you learn to focus on the inhaled breath and the exhaled breath, you experience a neutralizing effect on the mind. This reaction led Svatmarama to conclude that the control of *prana* is the key to super-awareness or *samadhi*.

In the chapter *Samadhi Prakarana* of the *Hathayoga Pradipika*, Svatmarama gives glimpses of his experiences of *samadhi*. He says, "If one learns not to think of external things and simultaneously keeps away inner thoughts, one experiences *samadhi*. When the mind is dissolved in the sea of the soul, an absolute state of existence is reached. This is *kaivalya*, the freedom of emancipation."

The goal of yoga is a state of equilibrium and peace. Patanjali warns the student of yoga not to be deceived by this quietness, for it could lead to a state of *yogabhrastha* or "falling from the grace of yoga". He also says, 'The practice of yoga must

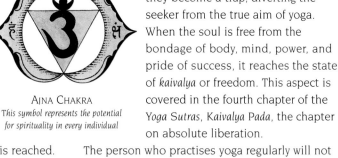

AJNA CHAKRA
This symbol represents the potential for spirituality in every individual

continue, as it has to culminate in the sight of the soul." This stage, when the individual becomes one with the core of his or her being, is a stage known as *nirbija* (seedless) *samadhi*.

IMPACT OF YOGA

In his third chapter of the *Yoga Sutras*, *Vibhuti Pada*, Patanjali speaks of the effects of yoga. Although they seem exotic to our modern conciousness, they indicate the potential of the powers of human nature. These spiritual powers and gifts have to be conquered in their turn. Otherwise, they become a trap, diverting the seeker from the true aim of yoga. When the soul is free from the bondage of body, mind, power, and pride of success, it reaches the state of *kaivalya* or freedom. This aspect is covered in the fourth chapter of the *Yoga Sutras*, *Kaivalya Pada*, the chapter on absolute liberation.

The person who practises yoga regularly will not become a victim but a master of his or her circumstances and time. The yoga practitioner lives to love and serve the world. This is the essence of life. Peace within and peace without, peace in the individual, in the family unit, in society, and in the world at large.

States of Mind

The mind is the vital link between the body and the consciousness. The individual can live with awareness, discrimination, and confidence only once the mind is calm and focused. Yoga is the alchemy that generates this equilibrium.

In yogic terminology, consciousness or *chitta* encompasses the mind or *manas*, intelligence or *buddhi*, and ego or *ahankara*. The Sanskrit word for man, *manusya* or *manava*, means "one who is endowed with this special consciousness". The mind does not have an actual location in the body. It is latent, elusive, and exists everywhere. The mind desires, wills, remembers, perceives, and experiences. Sensations of pain and pleasure, heat and cold, honour and dishonour, are experienced and interpreted by the mind. The mind reflects both the external and the internal worlds, but though it has the capacity to perceive things within and without, its natural tendency is to be preoccupied with the outside world.

NATURE OF THE MIND

When the mind is fully absorbed by objects seen, heard, smelled, felt, or tasted, this leads to stress, fatigue, and unhappiness. The mind can be a secret enemy and a treacherous friend. It influences our behaviour before we have the time to consider causes and consequences. Yoga trains the mind and inculcates a sense of discrimination, so that objects and events are seen for what they are and are not allowed to gain mastery over us.

FIVE MENTAL FACULTIES

We have five mental faculties which can be used in a positive or a negative way. These are: correct observation and knowledge, perception, imagination, dreamless sleep, and memory. Sometimes the mind loses its stability and clarity, and is either incapable of using its various faculties properly, or uses them in a negative way. The practice of yoga leads us to use these mental faculties in a positive way, thereby bringing the mind to a discriminative and attentive state. Awareness, together with discrimination and memory, target bad habits, which are essentially repetitive actions based on mistaken perception. These are then replaced by good habits. In this way, an individual becomes stronger, honest, and gains maturity. He or she is able to perceive and understand people, situations, and events with clarity. This seasoned, mature mind gradually transcends its frontiers to reach beyond mundane observation and experience, making the journey from confusion to clarity, one of the greatest benefits of yoga.

CLARITY OF MIND
Practising yoga gives you the ability to recognize situations for what they are, and to deal with them

"*The seasoned, mature mind transcends frontiers to reach beyond mundane observation.*"

DIFFERENT STATES OF MIND

Yogic science distinguishes between five basic states of mind. These are not grouped in stages, nor are they, except the last, unchangeable. According to Patanjali, these states of mind are: dull and lethargic, distracted, scattered, focused, and controlled. Patanjali described the lowest level of the mind as dull or *mudha*. A person in this state of mind is disinclined to observe, act, or react. This state is rarely inherent or permanent. It is usually caused by a traumatic experience, for instance, bereavement, or when a desired goal presents so many obstacles that the goal seems impossible to attain. After successive failures to take control of their lives, many people withdraw into dullness and lethargy. Often, this is exacerbated by either insomnia or oversleeping, comfort-eating, or the ingestion of tranquillizers and other substances which make the original problem worse. Yoga gradually transforms this feeling of defeat and helplessness into optimism and energy. The distracted state of mind is one where thoughts, feelings, and perceptions churn around in the consciousness, but leave no lasting impressions and hence serve no purpose. Patanjali calls this state, *ksipta*. Someone in a state of *ksipta* is unstable, unable to prioritize or focus on goals, usually because of flawed signals from the senses of perception he or she accepts and follows unthinkingly. This clouds the intellect and disturbs mental equilibrium. Such a state has to be calmed and brought to confront the factual knowledge of reality through the regular practice of yoga asanas and pranayama.

The most common state of mind is the scattered mind. In such a state, though the brain is active, it lacks purpose and direction. This state of mind is known as *viksipta*. Constantly plagued by doubt and fear, it alternates between decisiveness and lack of confidence. The regular practice of yoga gradually encourages the seeds of awareness and discrimination to take root, giving rise to a positive attitude and mental equilibrium.

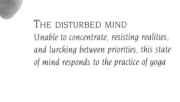

THE DISTURBED MIND
Unable to concentrate, resisting realities, and lurching between priorities, this state of mind responds to the practice of yoga

The ancient sages characterized the focused state of mind, or *ekagra*, as one that indicated a higher state of being. This is a liberated mind which has confronted afflictions and obstacles and conquered them. Such a mind has direction, concentration, and awareness. A person in this category of mental intelligence lives in the present without being caught in the past or future, undisturbed by external circumstances.

The fifth and highest state of mind is *niruddha*, or the controlled, restrained mind. According to Patanjali, *niruddha* is attained through the persistent practice of yoga, which allows an individual to conquer the lower levels of the mind.

At this level, the mind is linked exclusively with the object of its attention. It has the power to become totally absorbed in an activity, allowing nothing to disturb its absorption. When the brain is quiet, the intellect is at peace, the individual is serene and balanced, neither free nor bound, but poised in pure consciousness.

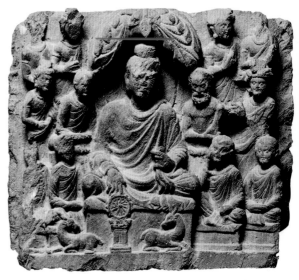

AN ENLIGHTENED MIND
The Buddha teaching his disciples the value of truth and contentment, from a frieze found at Sarnath, India

THE FINAL STAGE
The persistent practice of yoga allows you to conquer the lower levels of the mind and reach the peaks of self-realization

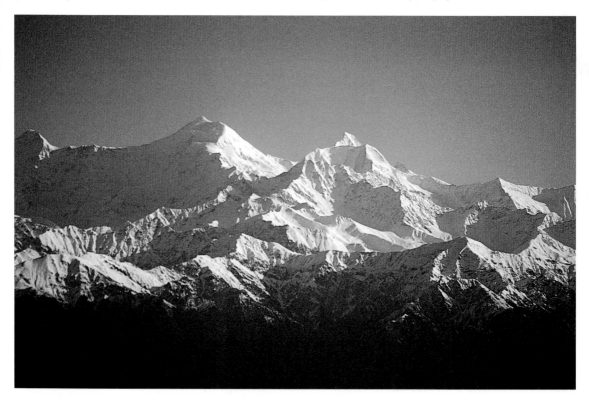

Eight Limbs

The basic tenets of yoga are described in the form of "eight limbs" or "steps" described by the sage, Patanjali. These are aphorisms, explaining the codes of ethical behaviour which will ultimately lead to self-realization.

The sage Patanjali reflected on the nature of man and the norms of society during his time. Then, very systematically, he expressed his observations in the form of aphorisms, which deal with the entire span of life, beginning with a code of correct conduct and ending with the ultimate goal, emancipation and freedom. These aphorisms outline the fundamental tenets of yoga, known as the eight limbs or *astanga*.

ASTANGA YOGA

The eight limbs or steps are *yama, niyama, asana, pranayama, pratyahara, dharana, dhyana,* and *samadhi*. These are sequential stages in an individual's life journey through yoga. Each step must be understood and followed to attain the ultimate goal of Astanga yoga, that of emancipation of the self. *Yama*, or general ethical principles, and *niyama*, or self-restraint, prescribe a code of conduct that moulds individual morality and behaviour. Asanas, or yogic poses, and pranayama, or breath control, discipline the body and the mind by basic practices conducive to physical, physiological, psychological, and mental health. Pranayama controls the mind, taming baser instincts, while *pratyahara*, or detachment from the

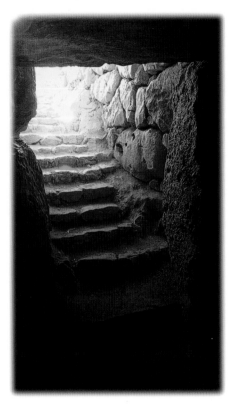

STEPS TO SELF-REALIZATION
Understand and absorb each stage to reach the ultimate goal

external world, stems the outgoing flow of the senses, withdrawing those of perception and the organs of action from worldly pleasures. *Dharana*, or concentration, guides the consciousness to focus attention rigorously on one point. *Dhyana*, or prolonged concentration, saturates the mind until it permeates to the source of existence, and the intellectual and conscious energy dissolves in the seat of the soul. It is then that *samadhi*, when you lose the sense of your separate existence, is attained. Nothing else remains except the core of one's being: the soul.

YAMA

Yama and *niyama* require tremendous inner discipline. *Yama* explains the codes of ethical behaviour to be observed and followed in everyday life, reminding us of our responsibilities as social beings. *Yama* has 5 principles. These are: *ahimsa* or non-violence, *satya* or truthfulness, *asteya* or freedom from avarice, *brahmacharya* or chastity, and *aparigraha* or freedom from desire. *Ahimsa* needs introspection to replace negative, destructive thoughts and actions by positive, constructive ones. Anger, cruelty, or harassment of others are facets of the violence latent in all of us.

These contradict the principles of *ahimsa*, while lying, cheating, dishonesty, and deception break the principles of *satya*. *Brahmacharya* does not mean total abstinence, but denotes a disciplined sexual life, promoting contentment and moral strength from within. *Parigraha* means "possession" or "covetousness", the instinct within all of us that traps us in the *karmic* cycle of reincarnation after death. However, while you may be able to give up material possessiveness, what about emotional or intellectual possessiveness? This is where Astanga yoga helps to discipline the mind, freeing it from the desire to possess, bringing it into a state of *aparigraha*, freedom from desire, as well as *asteya*, or freedom from greed.

NIYAMA
Niyama is the positive current that brings discipline, removes inertia, and gives shape to the inner desire to follow the yogic path. The principles of *niyama* are *saucha*, or cleanliness, *santosa*, or contentment, *tapas*, or austerity, *svadhyaya*, or the study of one's own self, which includes the body, mind, intellect, and ego. The final principle of *niyama* is *isvara pranidhana* or devotion to God. Contentment or *santosa* helps to curb desire, anger, ambition, and greed, while *tapas* or austerity involves self-discipline and the desire to purify the body, senses, and mind. The study and practice of yoga with devotional attention to the self and God is *tapas*.

ASANAS, PRANAYAMA, AND PRATYAHARA
According to the *Gheranda Samhita*, a text dating to the 15th century, written by the yogic sage, Gheranda: "The body soon decays like unbaked earthen pots thrown in water. Strengthen and purify

POSITIVE CURRENTS
Focus on your inner body and draw the mind inward

the body by baking it in the fire of yoga." Performing an asana helps to create and generate energy. Staying in an asana organizes and distributes this energy, while coming out of the pose protects the energy, preventing it from dissipating. In *Yoga Sutra* 111.47, Patanjali explains the effects of an asana as "*Rupa lavanya bala vajra samhananatvani kayasampat*". This means that a perfected body has beauty, grace, and strength which is comparable to the hardness and brilliance of a diamond. While practising an asana, one must focus attention on the inner body, drawing the mind inward to sharpen the intelligence.

Then, the asana becomes effortless as the blemishes on both the gross and the subtle body are washed off. This is the turning point in the practice of asanas, when the body, mind, and self unite. From this state begins the *isvara pranidhana*, or devotion to God. Asanas and pranayama are interrelated and inter-woven. Patanjali clearly specifies that pranayama should be attempted only after the asanas are mastered. *Prana* is "vital energy", which includes will power and ambition, while *ayama* means "stretch, expansion and extension". Pranayama can be described as the "expansion and extension of energy or life-force". Patanjali begins pranayama with the simple movement of breathing, leading us deeper and deeper into ourselves by teaching us to observe the very act of respiration. Pranayama has three movements – prolonged inhalation, deep exhalation, and prolonged, stable retention, all of which have to be performed with precision. Pranayama is the actual process of directing energy inward, making the mind fit for *pratyahara* or the detachment of the senses, which evolves from pranayama. When the senses withdraw from objects of desire, the mind is released from the power of the senses, which in turn become passive. Then the mind turns inward and is set free from the tyranny of the senses. This is *pratyahara*.

SAMYAMA – TOWARD THE LIBERATION OF THE SELF

Patanjali groups *dharana*, *dhyana*, and *samadhi* under the term *samyama* – the integration of the body, breath, mind, intellect, and self. It is not easy to explain the last three aspects of yoga as separate entities. The controlled mind that is gained in *pratyahara* is made to intensify its attention on a single thought in *dharana*. When this concentration is prolonged, it becomes *dhyana*. In *dhyana*, release,

expansion, quietness, and peace are experienced. This prolonged state of quietness frees an individual from attachment, resulting in indifference to the joys of pleasure or the sorrows of pain. The experience of *samadhi* is achieved when the knower, the knowable, and the known become one. When the object of meditation engulfs the meditator and becomes the subject, self-awareness is lost. This is *samadhi* – a state of total absorption. *Sama* means "level" or "alike", while *adhi* means "over" and "above". It also denotes the maintenance of the intelligence in a balanced state. Though *samadhi* can be explained at the intellectual level, it can only be experienced at the level of the heart. Ultimately, it is *samadhi* that is the fruit of the discipline of Astanga yoga.

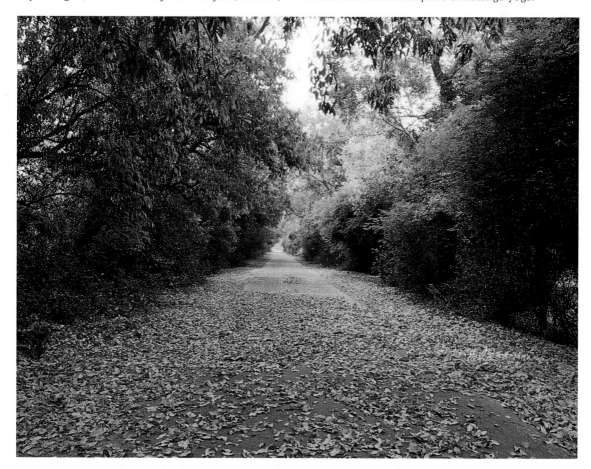

THE ROAD TO SAMADHI
The practice of yoga requires discipline and intense concentration, but the fruits of the journey are truth and tranquillity

Pranayama

Prana is the life-force which permeates both the individual as well as the universe at all levels. It is at once physical, sexual, mental, intellectual, spiritual, and cosmic. Prana, the breath, and the mind are inextricably linked to each other.

The ancient yogis advocated the practice of pranayama to unite the breath with the mind, and thus with the *prana* or life-force. *Prana* is energy, and *ayama* is the storing and distribution of that energy. *Ayama* has three aspects or movements: vertical extension, horizontal extension, and cyclical extension. By practising pranayama, we learn to move energy vertically, horizontally, and cyclically to the frontiers of the body.

Breath in pranayama

Pranayama is not deep breathing. Deep breathing tenses the facial muscles, makes the skull and scalp rigid, tightens the chest, and applies external force to the intake or release of breath. This creates hardness in the fibres of the lungs and chest, preventing the percolation of breath through the body.

In pranayama, the cells of the brain and the facial muscles remain soft and receptive, and the breath is drawn in or released gently. During inhalation, each molecule, fibre, and cell of the body is independently felt by the mind, and is allowed to receive and absorb the *prana*. There are no sudden movements and one becomes aware of the gradual expansion of the respiratory organs, and feels the breath reaching the remotest parts of the lungs.

In exhalation, the release of breath is gradual, and this gives the air cells sufficient time to re-absorb the residual *prana* to the maximum possible extent. This allows for the full utilization of energy, thus building up emotional stability and calming the mind.

The practice of asanas removes the obstructions which impede the flow of *prana*. During pranayama, one should be totally absorbed in the fineness of inhalation, exhalation, and in the naturalness of retention. One should not disturb or jerk the vital organs and nerves, or stress the brain cells. The brain is the instrument which observes the smooth flow of inhalation and exhalation. One must be aware of the interruptions which occur during a single inhalation and exhalation.

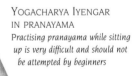

YOGACHARYA IYENGAR
IN PRANAYAMA
Practising pranayama while sitting up is very difficult and should not be attempted by beginners

Check these, and a smooth flow will set in. Similarly, during retention of breath, learn to retain the first indrawn breath with stability. If this stability is lost, it is better to release the breath, rather than strain to hold it. While inhaling or retaining the breath in a pranayamic cycle, remember to ensure that the abdomen does not swell.

THE FINAL GOAL

Attempt pranayama only when the yoga asanas have been mastered. Patanjali reiterates this several times, most emphatically in *Yoga Sutra* II, 49. The next *sutra*, *Yoga Sutra* II, 50, explains that inhalation, exhalation, and retention must be precise. The *sutra* begins with control over the movement of exhalation, or *bahya*, and inhalation, or *abhyantara*. Each inhalation activates the central nervous system into stimulating the peripheral nerves, and each exhalation triggers the reverse process. During the retention of breath, both processes take place. The *Hathayoga Pradipika* speaks of *antara-kumbhaka* and *bahya-kumbhaka*, or the suspension of breath with full or empty lungs, as well as inhalation, and exhalation. Pranayama is a complex process composed of all these. It has to be practised with the greatest sincerity and precision. You cannot achieve pranayama just because you want to – you have to be ready for it.

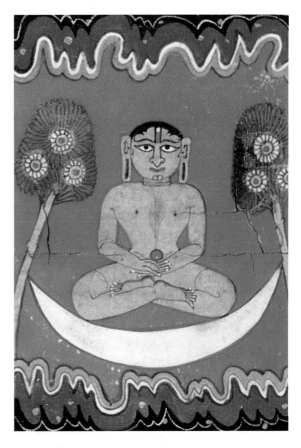

A YOGI IN PRANAYAMA
For more than a thousand years, sages have practised pranayama, controlling their breath and with it, their mind

ANCIENT TRADITIONS
An illustrated folio from the Kalpasutra, 15th-century texts describing the path to health and spirituality

PRANAYAMA

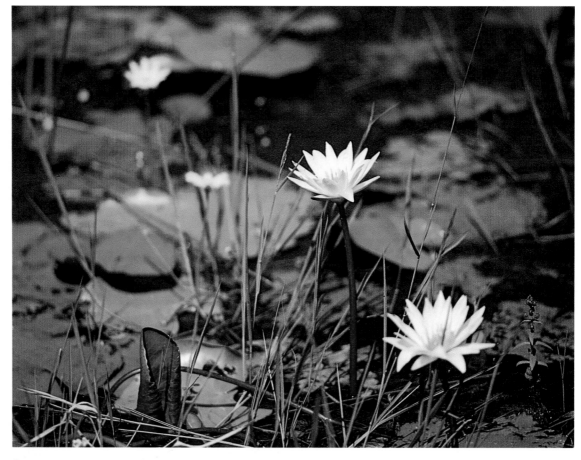

SPIRITUAL PRANAYAMA
The pranayamic mind blossoms, becomes completely free, and dissolves in the self

In pranayamic breathing, the brain is quiet, and this allows the nervous system to function more effectively. Inhalation is the art of receiving primeval energy into the body in the form of breath, and bringing the spiritual cosmic breath into contact with the individual breath. Exhalation is the removal of toxins from the system.

BETWEEN THE MATERIAL AND SPIRITUAL WORLD
Pranayama is also the link between the physiological and spiritual organisms of man. At first, pranayama is difficult and requires great effort. Mastery is achieved when pranayama becomes effortless. Just as the diaphragm is the meeting point of the physiological and spiritual body, the retention of

energy or *kumbhaka* is realizing the very core of your body. Once the external movements are controlled, there is internal silence. In such a silence there is no thought as the mind has then dissolved in the self.

In the *Hathayoga Pradipika*, the sage Svatmarama gives a detailed description of the ways in which an individual comes to experience the elevated state of oneness with the self through the practice of pranayama. Hence, practising it is not only very difficult, but also highly absorbing. If you fail after a few cycles, be content with the knowledge that you have practised three or four cycles with awareness and attention. Do not turn away from failures. Accept them and learn from them. Gradually, you will learn to master pranayama.

Chakras

Yogic science recognizes that spiritual health is activated by a system of chakras or "nerve" centres, said to be located within the spinal column. Cosmic energy lies coiled within these chakras and has to be awakened for self-realization.

Modern technology has provided us with the means to examine the state of our bodies. But nothing has helped us discern character, personality, or the potential for goodness. The most important aspect of a human being is the part which lies between the outer skin and the innermost soul – the *shakti*, which includes the mind, intellect, emotions, vital energy, the sense of "I", the powers of will and discrimination, and the conscience. These are different in every human being, and that makes us individually both mysterious and unique.

In yogic terminology, the soul is called *purusha shakti*, while *prakriti shakti* or the energy of nature, came to be called *kundalini* by the ancient yogis.

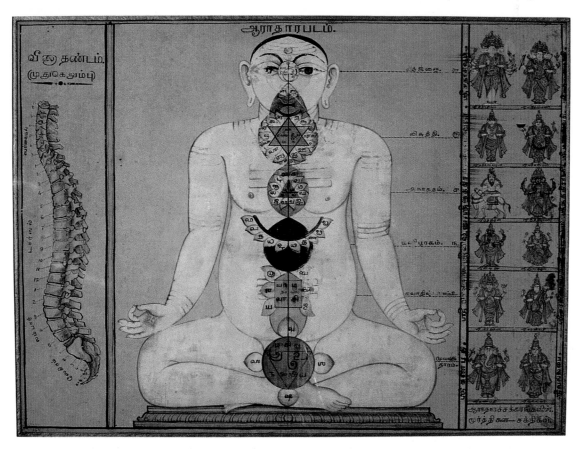

THE 7 MAIN CHAKRAS OF THE BODY
Yogic sages believed chakras were located along the spinal column

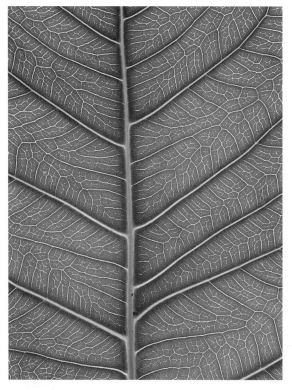

EACH CELL IS AN ENTITY
Energy spreads through a leaf, from each tiny cell connected to the other, permeating from the stalks to the entire plant

We have always known that health is important, but it is time to realize, as proponents of yoga have known for generations, that our physical condition is inextricably linked to our state of mind.

Yogic science recognized this connection from the very beginning. In order to achieve perfect physical health, the ancient sages concluded, you must activate the body's *chakras*. *Chakras* are notionally located along the spine, from the brain to the tailbone. But while the spine is a physical entity, *chakras* are not composed of matter. Although they possess no physicality, they govern all the elements of the body.

THE MEANING OF CHAKRAS

Chakra means "wheel" or "ring" in Sanskrit and our personal *chakras* have energy coiled within them. They are the critical junctions which determine the state of the body and mind. Just as the brain controls physical, mental, and intellectual functions through the nerve cells or neurons, *chakras* tap the *prana* or cosmic energy which is within all living beings and transform it into spiritual energy. This is spread through the body by the *nadis*, or channels.

Being invisible, *chakras* are tangible only through their effects. They can be accessed once the student of yoga has achieved all the eight aspects of yoga (*see page 29*), when the human self merges with the divine self.

Kundalini is the divine, cosmic energy which exists as a latent force in everyone. When the *prakriti shakti* is awakened, it gravitates toward the very core of the soul or *purusha shakti*.

AWAKENING COSMIC ENERGY

This fire of divine, cosmic energy is ignited by *yoga-agni*, the fire of yoga. When a fire is covered with ashes, it goes out. In the same way, if our senses are inert, or if we are motivated by pride, self-indulgence, and envy, the *kundalini* is kept in a dormant state. If we allow such negative qualities to dominate our thinking over long periods, our spiritual evolution is not merely hampered, but actually halted.

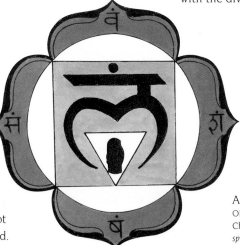

A SYMBOLIC REPRESENTATION OF THE MULADHARA CHAKRA
Chakras transform cosmic energy into spiritual energy

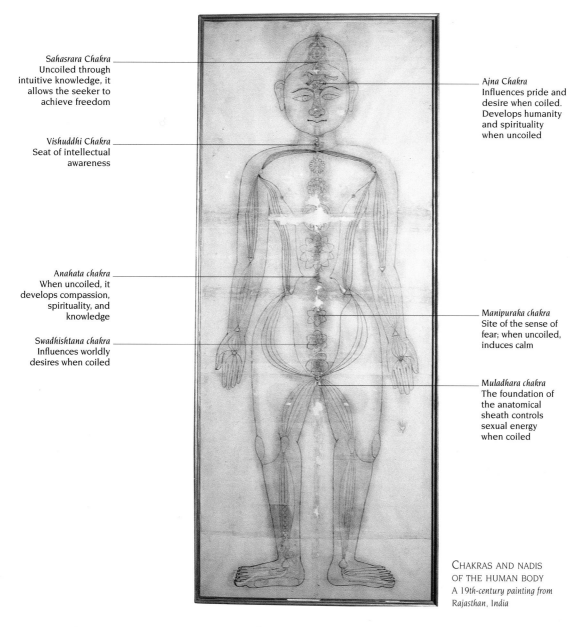

Sahasrara Chakra
Uncoiled through intuitive knowledge, it allows the seeker to achieve freedom

Vishuddhi Chakra
Seat of intellectual awareness

Anahata chakra
When uncoiled, it develops compassion, spirituality, and knowledge

Swadhishtana chakra
Influences worldly desires when coiled

Ajna Chakra
Influences pride and desire when coiled. Develops humanity and spirituality when uncoiled

Manipuraka chakra
Site of the sense of fear; when uncoiled, induces calm

Muladhara chakra
The foundation of the anatomical sheath controls sexual energy when coiled

CHAKRAS AND NADIS OF THE HUMAN BODY
A 19th-century painting from Rajasthan, India

There are 11 *chakras* of which 7 are crucial (*see diagram above*), and the others dependent. The most important is the Sahasrara *chakra*, where *prakriti shakti* or energy, unites with *purusha shakti*, or soul.

The practice of yoga is directed at awakening the divine energy within every human being. Asanas and pranayama uncoil and alert the *chakras*. In the process, the *nadis* are activated. This causes the *chakras* to vibrate and to generate energy, which is then circulated all over the body through the *nadis*. The emotions rooted in the *chakras* are transformed as divine energy is awakened and circulated.

To achieve self-realization the sincere student of yoga will, with persistent, rigorous practice, conquer the 6 main obstacles to happiness – desire, anger, greed, infatuation, pride, and envy.

The Guru & the Yogi

*The tradition of the guru, or master, and the yogi, or disciple, is an ancient one. All
learning from generation to generation has been handed down this way. The guru
must be compassionate, yet exacting. The yogi must be sincere and dedicated.*

How do we distinguish between the true guru and the false one? The cult of the guru, or master, is an Asian concept. To other societies, the concept might seem exotic, mysterious, or even abhorrent – a brake on individual freedom or judgment. Some thinkers have declared that a guru is not needed at all, while others believe that you cannot reach your goal without one. Perhaps the importance of the guru can be explained by examining its Sanskrit root. *Gu* means "darkness" and *ru* means "light" – therefore, a guru is one who leads you from darkness to light. Although the *sadhaka* or seeker has to tread the spiritual path to self-realization alone, the guru's guidance is essential to show the right path and to safeguard the yogi, the student of yoga, who decides to follow it.

AN ANCIENT TRADITION

The guru is the voice of consciousness during the process of spiritual awakening. In India, the relationship between a guru and a disciple is an ancient tradition, and has been the foundation of all learning. The *guru-sishya parampara* (*sishya* means "disciple" and *parampara* means "tradition") has been the system through which knowledge has been handed down, generation to generation and age to age. The energy that the guru has imbibed from *his* teacher is passed on to his disciple, keeping the process of communication alive from one epoch to the next. The guru opens the disciple's eyes to awareness. Knowledge exists, but ignorance veils it,

YOGACHARYA IYENGAR WITH A STUDENT
The guru does not only teach asanas, he teaches you how to live

and it is the guru who removes this veil from the intellect of the *sishya*. The guru is the guide who opens the gate of the student's dormant faculties and awakens the latent power and energy within. Being with the guru is like being in the sunlight, and the glow lasts for eternity.

The relationship between the teacher and the disciple is a unique one. It is similar, but not identical, to a mother and child. Just as a mother loves, nourishes, guides, cajoles into obedience, rebukes, educates, and protects her child, the guru takes the disciple into his care, making it his life's work to mould his student into perfect shape, physically, mentally, and spiritually.

THE GURU

Yoga is a discipline and the yogic texts aptly begin with the emphasis on discipline or *anusasanam*: "Without discipline, nothing can be achieved." The guru does not enforce discipline with strictness, but builds up an awareness of it in his student, allowing the latter to develop inner discipline. A wise guru does not lay down codes of conduct, but motivates the disciple by precept and example.

The guru does not demand attention, he commands it. In the process of teaching, he creates total confidence in the disciple, and helps him or her develop the will power to face all circumstances with equanimity. The guru constantly improves on his teaching techniques, opening the disciple's eyes, improvising where necessary to create new dimensions in his teaching. The guru is compassionate, but does not expect emotional attachment from his disciple, nor does he become emotionally attached himself.

The guru should be confident, challenging, caring, cautious, constructive, and courageous. The clarity and creativity of his teaching should reflect his devotion and dedication to his subject – in this case, the complexities and subtleties of yoga.

THE DISCIPLE

An ideal disciple is obedient, earnest, serious, and always ready to follow the teachings of his or her guru. This is not unthinking obedience, but one based on respect and a sincere desire to learn. Disciples can be dull, average, or superior. The dull student has little enthusiasm, is unstable, timorous, and self-indulgent. He or she is unwilling to put in the hard work required which is needed to attain the goal of self-realization.

The average student is indecisive, attracted equally to worldly pleasures as to spiritual matters.

While conscious of the highest good, this student lacks the determination to persevere, and is unable to hold on steadfastly to the yogic path. He or she needs firmness and discipline from his or her guru, a fact the guru recognizes at once.

The superior or intense student, on the other hand, has vision, enthusiasm, and courage. He or she resists temptations and does not hesitate to cast off qualities that distract him or her from the goal. This student becomes steady, stable, and skilful. The guru guides this kind of student to the ultimate goal of self-realization.

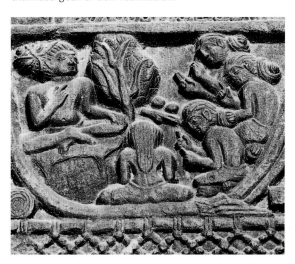

A SAGE TEACHING HIS PUPILS
This 2nd-century BC frieze from Bharhut, India, points to the antiquity of the guru-yogi tradition

While practising yoga, the disciple must recall and deliberate on each word and action of the guru and consolidate each learning experience. Today's disciple may become the guru of tomorrow. Clarity of mind and firmness of resolve to tread the path to self-realization is essential. The yogi must have *riti* and *niti* – method and morality – to impart to the disciple, the learning, the experience, and wisdom gleaned over the years. Thus, the tradition of the guru and the yogi is carried on for yet another generation.

This book is my attempt to disseminate my knowledge of yoga to all those across the world who wish to become true followers of yoga.

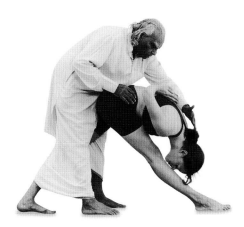

CHAPTER 3

"The body is your temple. Keep it pure and clean for the soul to reside in."

Asanas for You

The science of yoga is like the art of music. There is a rhythm within the body, and that can only be maintained by paying attention to each step of the asana, and to the progression between asanas. In your practice of yoga, there has to be a physical, physiological, psychological, and spiritual rhythm. Unless there is harmony and melody, the music will not be worth listening to. The body is a truly sensitive and receptive instrument, and its vibrations, like sound, express the harmony or dissonance within it. Each of these vibrations must synchronize in the movement, which is the asana.

Classic Poses

Yoga asanas cover the basic positions of standing, sitting, forward bends, twists, inversions, back bends, and lying down. The classic poses must be practised with physical co-ordination, as well as intelligence and sincerity.

There is more to practising asanas correctly than merely the physical aligning of the body. The classic poses, when practised with discrimination and awareness, bring the body, mind, intelligence, nerves, consciousness, and the self together into a single, harmonious whole. Asanas may appear to deal with the physical body alone but, in fact, different asanas can affect the chemical messages sent to and from the brain, improving and stabilizing your mental state. Yoga's unique ability to soothe the nerves – the medium between the physiological body and the psychological body – calms the brain, makes the mind fresh and tranquil, and relaxes the entire body.

I have selected these asanas because they cover all the basic positions of yoga: standing, sitting, forward bends, twists, inversions, back bends, and lying down. The regular practice of these asanas, stimulates and activates all the organs, tissues,

and cells of the body. The mind becomes alert and strong, the body healthy and active.

The anatomical body comprises the limbs and the actual parts of the body. The physical body is made up of bones, muscles, skin, and tissue. The physiological body is composed of the heart, lungs, liver, spleen, pancreas, intestines, and the other organs. The nerves, brain, and intellect make up the psychological body. To practise asanas correctly, you have to learn to bring all these levels together.

STAGES OF LEARNING YOGA

Newcomers to yoga approach asanas with "uncultured" minds. They have to learn that at first asanas are practised at the level of the anatomical body alone – the stage called *arambhavastha*. This beginner's stage is important and should not be hurried through. In order to learn the asanas, beginners should be primarily concerned with getting their movements right. In the step-by-step instructions to the asanas in this chapter, I have highlighted the points you should concentrate on, the important motions and movements in the pose you need to take note of. Beginners have to grasp the whole asana, and not lose themselves in the finer details. It is more important for you to start by striving for stability within a pose. This provides a strong foundation. You will then enter the intermediate stage, or *ghatavastha*, in which the mind is affected by changes in the body. When you reach this stage, you are practising the movements correctly, your body is under

INTEGRATING BODY AND SPIRIT
Yogacharya Iyengar in
Adhomukha Svanasana

"*Asanas keep your body, as well as your mind, healthy and active.*"

your control, but you must now push your mind to touch every part of your body. In my instructions to the asanas in this chapter, I have pointed out that students of yoga at this stage must practise the asanas with reflective and meditative attention. You must become aware of your tissues, organs, skin, and even individual cells. Your mind must flow along with all of these parts.

Parichayavastha, or the advanced stage, comes next. This is the stage of intimate knowledge, when your mind brings your body in touch with your intelligence. Once this happens, the mind ceases to be a separate entity, and the intelligence and the body become one. I have included the concepts that the advanced practitioner of yoga should focus on. Your adjustments are more subtle and discriminating now, and are in the realm of the mental and physiological body, rather than merely in your muscles, bones, and joints. The final stage, *nishpattyavastha*, is the state of perfection. Once the intelligence feels the oneness between the flesh and the skin, it introduces the *atman* – the self or soul. This frees the body and integrates it with the soul in the journey from the finite to the infinite. Then the body, mind, and self become one. At this stage, asanas become meditative and spiritual. This may be termed "dynamic meditation".

WHAT IS AN ASANA?
An asana is not a posture that you assume mechanically. It involves a thoughtful process at the end of which a balance is achieved between movement and resistance. Your weight has to be evenly distributed over muscles, bones, and

joints, just as your intelligence must be engaged at every level. You have to create space in your muscles and your skin, fitting the fine network of your entire body into the asana. This helps the organs of perception (the eyes, ears, nose, tongue, and skin) to discern the subtlety of each movement. This conjunction between the organs of action and organs of perception occurs when the student reaches a subjective understanding of an asana, and begins, through instinct as well as knowledge, to adjust his or her movements correctly. Practise with dedication. Be completely absorbed by the asana.

Once both sides of the body become symmetrical, undue stress is removed from the circulatory, respiratory, digestive, reproductive, and excretory systems. In each asana, different organs are placed in different anatomical positions, and are squeezed and spread, dampened and dried, heated and cooled. The organs are supplied with fresh blood, and are gently massaged, relaxed, and toned into a state of optimum health.

MOVEMENT AND RESISTANCE
The final pose of Utthita Parsvakonasana

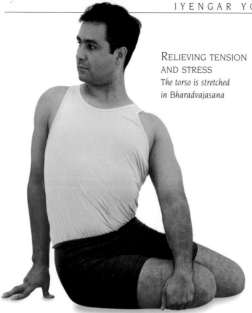

RELIEVING TENSION
AND STRESS
*The torso is stretched
in Bharadvajasana*

CLASSIC POSES

SITTING ASANAS

All sitting asanas bring elasticity to the hips, knees, ankles, and muscles of the groin. These poses remove tension and hardness in the diaphragm and throat, making breathing smoother and easier. They keep the spine steady, pacifying the mind and stretching the muscles of the heart. Blood circulation increases to all parts of the body.

STANDING ASANAS

Standing asanas strengthen the leg muscles and joints, and increase the suppleness and strength of the spine. Owing to their rotational and flexing movements, the spinal muscles and inter-vertebral joints are kept mobile and well-aligned. The arteries of the legs are stretched, increasing the blood supply to the lower limbs, and preventing thrombosis in the calf muscles. These asanas also tone the cardio-vascular system. The lateral wall of the heart is fully stretched, increasing the supply of fresh blood to the heart.

FORWARD BENDS

In forward bends, the abdominal organs are compressed. This has a unique effect on the nervous system: as these organs relax, the frontal brain is cooled, and the flow of blood to the entire brain is regulated. The sympathetic nervous system is rested, bringing down the pulse rate and blood pressure. Stress is removed from the organs of perception and the senses relax. The adrenal glands are also soothed and function more efficiently. Since the body is in a horizontal position in forward bends, the heart is relieved of the strain of pumping blood against gravity, and blood circulates through all parts of the body easily. Forward bends also strengthen the paraspinal muscles, inter-vertebral joints, and ligaments.

TWISTS

These asanas teach us the importance of a healthy spine and inner body. In twists, the pelvic and abdominal organs are squeezed and flushed with blood. They improve the suppleness of the diaphragm, and relieve spinal, hip, and groin disorders. The spine also becomes more supple, and this improves the flow of blood to the spinal nerves and increases energy levels.

INVERSIONS

Some people fear that if they practise inverted poses, their blood pressure will rise, or their blood vessels burst. These are complete misconceptions. After all, standing for long periods can lead to thrombosis and varicose veins, but no one is going to stop standing up! Standing upright is a result of evolution. Just as the human body has adjusted to an upright position, it can also learn to perform inversions without any risk or harm. In contrast to the twisting asanas, inverted asanas have a drying effect on the pelvic and abdominal organs, while vital organs like the brain, heart, and lungs are flushed with blood. According to the third chapter of the sage Svatmarama's *Hathayoga Pradipika,*

Salamba Sirsasana (headstand, *see page* 118) is the king of asanas, and Salamba Sarvangasana (shoulderstand, *see page* 124) the queen of asanas. The health of your body and mind is greatly enhanced by the practice of these two asanas.

BACK BENDS

All back bends stimulate the central nervous system and increase its ability to bear stress. They help to relieve one from stress, tension, and nervous exhaustion. These asanas stimulate and energize the body, and are invaluable to people suffering from depression. In Urdhva Dhanurasana (*see page* 140) the liver and spleen are fully stretched, and can therefore function more effectively.

RECLINING ASANAS

Reclining asanas are restful poses which soothe the body and refresh the mind. While reclining asanas are often sequenced at the end of a yoga session, they are also preparatory asanas, as they help relax the body and strengthen the joints. They give the body the required energy for the more strenuous asanas. Savasana (*see page* 150), for instance, helps to recover the breath and cool the body and the mind. Reclining asanas prepare you for pranayama.

PRACTISING CLASSIC POSES

Practise classic poses when you feel confident of the suppleness of your body and the stability of your mind. I recommend that beginners and those with stiff muscles or joints, or people with specific ailments, might prefer to practise with props for the first 6-8 months. If you normally practise classic poses without props, you may, however, wish to use them on days when you are feeling tired, or if a particular part of your body feels stiff. For information on props, and how to use them, see *Yoga: The Path to Holistic Health*, by B.K.S Iyengar (Dorling Kindersley, 2001).

STRETCHING OUT
Paschimottanasana extends the spine

Always sequence your asanas with care. Whenever you practise, take care not to "harden" your brain. This occurs when you hold your breath, and your head becomes tense and heavy, particularly common when practising standing asanas and forward bends. This can also happen in a standing asana when you use force to descend without fully extending your spine. Since the action is achieved by force, rather than by utilizing the intelligence of the spine, this results in tension in the spine. I call this situation "hardening the brain" because it means you are not allowing your brain to be sufficiently sensitive to your body's actions. Similarly, in back bends, if force, not intelligence is applied while extending the back, the cervical region remains hard. This, too, "hardens the brain".

"BRAIN" OF THE POSE

In each asana, a specific part of your body is the "brain" of the pose. For instance, the outstretched arm is the "brain" of Utthita Parsvakonasana (*see page* 60), the centre of balance in the pose. When you practise, observe this specific part of your body carefully and focus on it. Bring a firmness and steadiness to it. This will then spread to the rest of your body and bring it under your control. Gradually, you will be able to experience the pose at the physiological, and not merely the physical level.

PRACTICE WITHOUT FEAR
Inversions, like Salamba Sarvangasana, are good for your body and mind

Standing Asanas

*"An asana is not a posture which
you assume mechanically.
It involves thought, at the end
of which a balance is achieved
between movement
and resistance."*

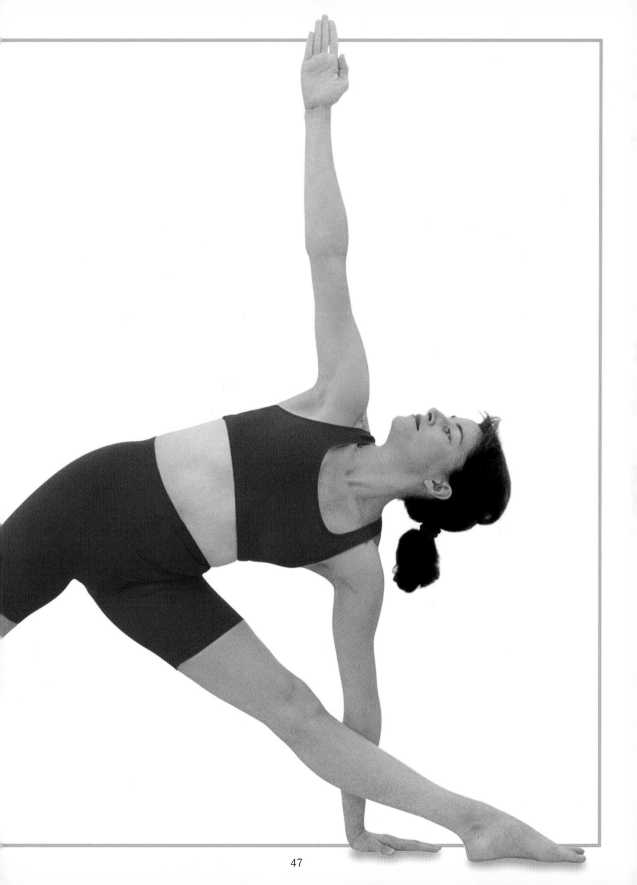

ताडासन

Tadasana

- Mountain posture -

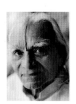

IN THIS POSTURE you learn to stand as firm and erect as a mountain. The word *tada* in Sanskrit means "mountain". Most people do not balance perfectly on both legs, leading to ailments which can be avoided. Tadasana teaches you the art of standing correctly and increases your awareness of your body. It is the foundation stone for other asanas. Practising it gives rise to a sense of firmness, strength, stillness, and steadiness.

CAUTIONS
◆

If you have Parkinson's disease or a spinal disc disorder, you may find it helpful to stand facing a wall with your palms placed on it. People with scoliosis should rest the spine against the protruding edge of two adjoining walls.

Keep the head, neck, and spine in a straight line

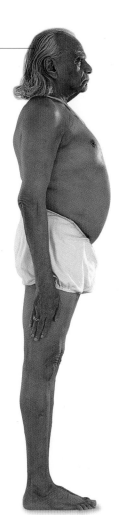

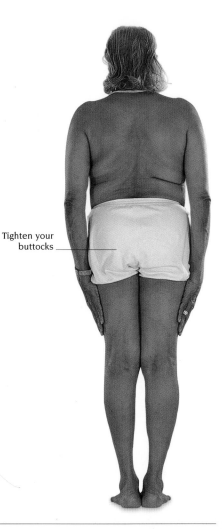

Tighten your buttocks

1 Stand with your feet together on a smooth, uncovered floor. Make sure that your feet are in line with each other, with both the big toes and heels touching. If you find it difficult to keep your feet together, separate them by about 7cm (2-3in). Rest your weight on the centres of the arches of the feet. Keep the heels firm and toes extended. Stretch out your toes and keep them relaxed.

2 Press your feet firmly down on the floor and stretch both your legs upward. Keep both ankles in line with each other. Your legs should be perpendicular to the floor and aligned to each other. Tighten your kneecaps and quadriceps and pull them upward. Draw your hips inward by compressing them as well as your buttocks.

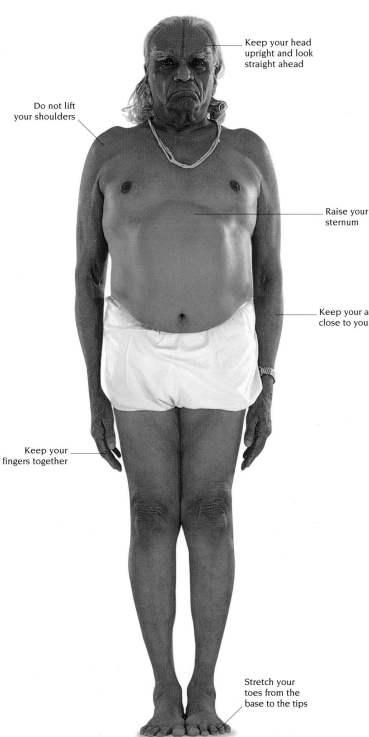

Keep your head upright and look straight ahead

Do not lift your shoulders

Raise your sternum

Keep your arms close to your sides

Keep your fingers together

Stretch your toes from the base to the tips

BENEFITS

◆

Corrects bad posture by straightening the spine

◆

Improves the alignment of your body

◆

Counters the degenerative effects of ageing on the spine, legs, and feet

◆

Tones the buttock muscles

3 Extend your arms along the sides of your body, with your palms facing your thighs and fingers pointing down. Keep the head and spine in a straight line. Stretch your neck without tensing the muscles. Pull your lower abdomen in and up. Lift your sternum and broaden your chest. Breathe normally during all the steps of the asana.

4 Press your heels, as well as the mounds of your toes down on the floor. This will place equal pressure on the outer and inner edges of the feet. Guard against balancing on the front of the feet. Now, consciously rest most of your weight on your heels. Hold the pose for 20-30 seconds.

उत्थित त्रिकोणासन

Utthita Trikonasana

- Extended triangle pose -

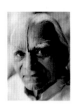

IN THIS ASANA, your body takes the shape of an extended triangle, giving an intense stretch to your trunk and legs. *Utthita* means "extended" in Sanskrit, *tri* means "three", and *kona* indicates an angle. With practice, you will learn to move from your physical body into your physiological body (*see page* 42). You will learn to activate the organs, glands, and nerves – which form the physiological body – by controlling the movements of your limbs. This pose tones the ligaments and improves flexibility.

CAUTIONS
◆

If you are prone to dizzy spells, vertigo, or high blood pressure, look down at the floor in the final pose. Do not turn your head up. If you have a cardiac condition, practise against a wall. Do not raise the arm, but rest it along your hip.

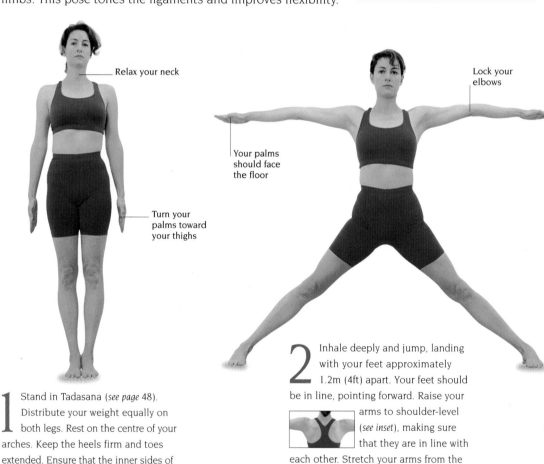

Relax your neck

Lock your elbows

Your palms should face the floor

Turn your palms toward your thighs

1 Stand in Tadasana (*see page* 48). Distribute your weight equally on both legs. Rest on the centre of your arches. Keep the heels firm and toes extended. Ensure that the inner sides of both feet touch each other. Keep your back straight. Breathe evenly.

2 Inhale deeply and jump, landing with your feet approximately 1.2m (4ft) apart. Your feet should be in line, pointing forward. Raise your arms to shoulder-level (*see inset*), making sure that they are in line with each other. Stretch your arms from the back of your elbows. Lift your chest and look straight ahead.

3 Turn your right foot in slightly to the left, maintaining the stretch of your other leg. Then, turn your left foot 90° to the left, keeping the right leg stretched and tightened at the knee. Make sure that your arms do not waver. Keep them fully stretched.

NOTE To maintain your balance during this step, always keep to the sequence of turning in your right foot first. Once you have done this, turn your left foot out.

ADVANCED BEGINNERS For a better stretch in the final pose, press your

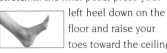 left heel down on the floor and raise your toes toward the ceiling (*see inset*). Then tighten the left knee and flatten your foot to the floor again.

CORRECTING YOURSELF

   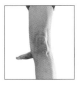

THE RIGHT KNEE

WRONG If your right knee rotates to the right, this will impair your stretch in the final pose.

RIGHT Keep your right kneecap facing front. Ensure that your right thigh does not turn inward.

THE LEFT KNEE

WRONG If the left knee rotates too far to the left, your balance in the final pose will be affected.

RIGHT Keep your left knee tightened, and in line with the centre of your left foot, shin, and thigh.

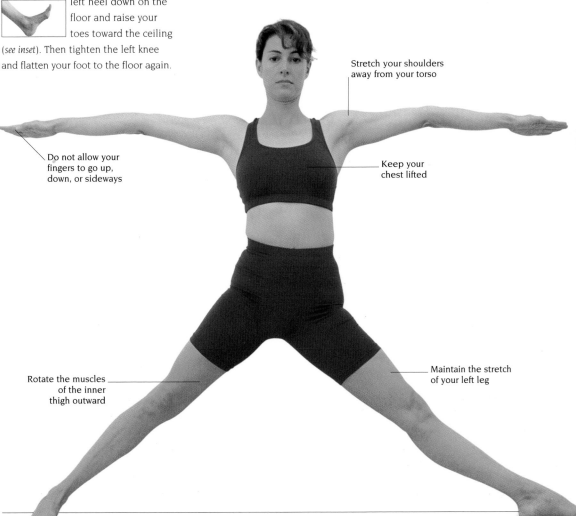

Stretch your shoulders away from your torso

Do not allow your fingers to go up, down, or sideways

Keep your chest lifted

Rotate the muscles of the inner thigh outward

Maintain the stretch of your left leg

उत्थित त्रिकोणासन

Utthita Trikonasana

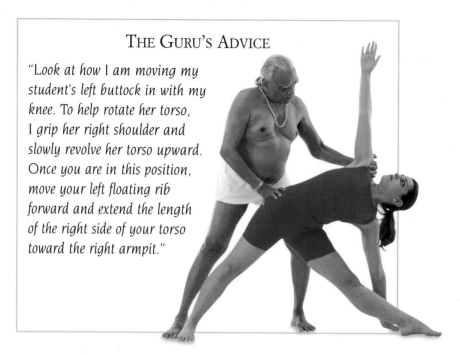

THE GURU'S ADVICE

"Look at how I am moving my student's left buttock in with my knee. To help rotate her torso, I grip her right shoulder and slowly revolve her torso upward. Once you are in this position, move your left floating rib forward and extend the length of the right side of your torso toward the right armpit."

CORRECTING YOURSELF

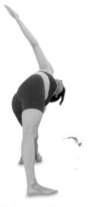

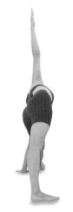

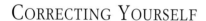

WRONG If your right arm tilts back, you will lose the correct alignment of the hips and buttocks. Your neck and head will jut forward and your weight will fall on your left palm, and not on your left heel.

RIGHT The right arm is stretched straight upward from the armpit and kept steady. Keep the back of your head aligned to your spine, and keep your shoulder blades in line with each other.

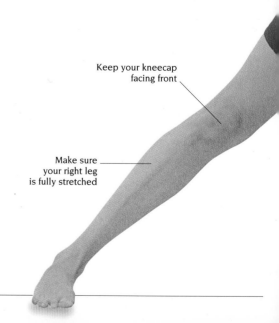

Keep your kneecap facing front

Make sure your right leg is fully stretched

4 Exhale, and bend your torso sideways to the left. Place your left palm flat on the floor, and press your left heel down on the floor. Adjust your pose until your weight rests on your left heel and not on your left palm. Raise your right arm up toward the ceiling, in line with your shoulders and left arm. Turn your head, keeping your neck passive, and fix your eyes on your right thumb. Stay in the pose for 20-30 seconds. Do not take deep breaths, but breathe evenly.

NOTE If you feel unsteady, when you bend, first grip your left ankle with your left hand. Bring the left buttock forward slightly. Place your right hand on your right hip. Once you feel steady, follow the instructions above.

BENEFITS

Relieves gastritis, indigestion, acidity, and flatulence

◆

Improves the flexibility of the spine

◆

Alleviates backache

◆

Corrects alignment of the shoulders

◆

Helps to treat neck sprains

◆

Massages and tones the pelvic area

◆

Strengthens the ankles

◆

Reduces discomfort during menstruation

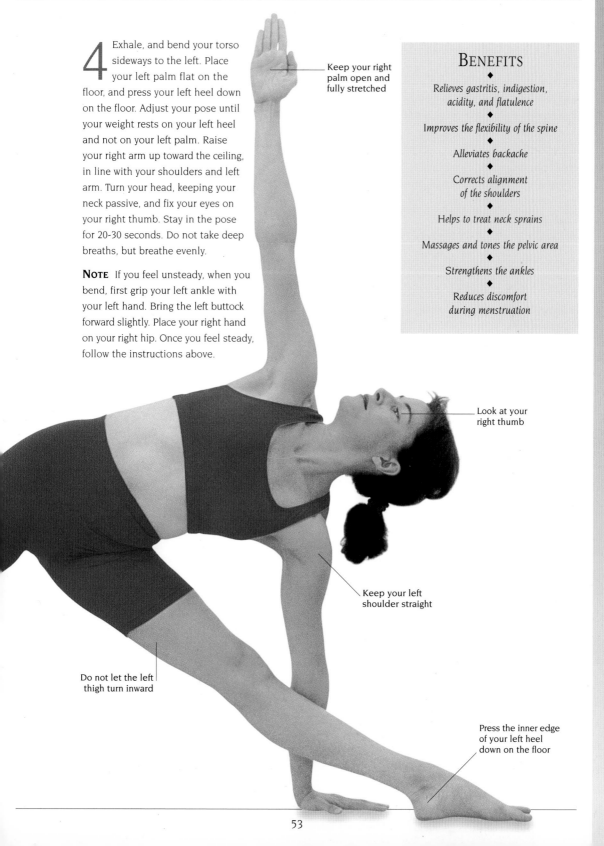

Keep your right palm open and fully stretched

Look at your right thumb

Keep your left shoulder straight

Do not let the left thigh turn inward

Press the inner edge of your left heel down on the floor

उत्थित त्रिकोणासन

Utthita Trikonasana

ADVANCED WORK IN THE POSE

Keep your right arm steady, as it is the "brain" of the pose (*see page* 45). Work on your back. Imagine your body is being pulled in opposite directions from the spine. Check that both shoulders are equally stretched out. Make sure that your torso revolves slightly upward and back. Keep the back of your neck in line with your spine – but relax your throat, keeping the muscles of your neck passive. Ensure that your tailbone and the back of your head align with each other, and that your whole body is balanced symmetrically in one plane.

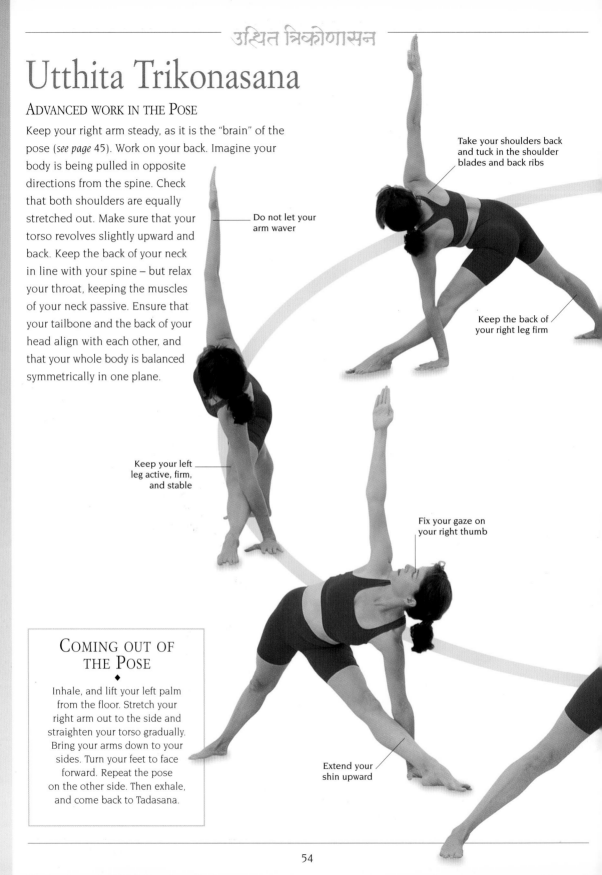

Do not let your arm waver

Keep your left leg active, firm, and stable

Take your shoulders back and tuck in the shoulder blades and back ribs

Keep the back of your right leg firm

Fix your gaze on your right thumb

Extend your shin upward

COMING OUT OF THE POSE

◆

Inhale, and lift your left palm from the floor. Stretch your right arm out to the side and straighten your torso gradually. Bring your arms down to your sides. Turn your feet to face forward. Repeat the pose on the other side. Then exhale, and come back to Tadasana.

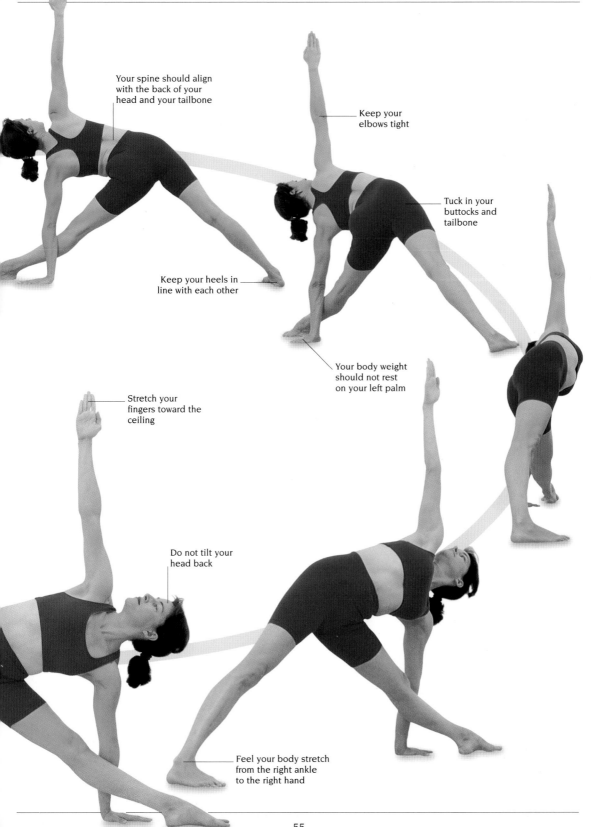

Your spine should align with the back of your head and your tailbone

Keep your elbows tight

Tuck in your buttocks and tailbone

Keep your heels in line with each other

Your body weight should not rest on your left palm

Stretch your fingers toward the ceiling

Do not tilt your head back

Feel your body stretch from the right ankle to the right hand

वीरभद्रासन २
Virabhadrasana 2

- Warrior pose 2 -

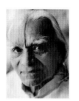

THIS POSE IS NAMED after Virabhadra, a legendary warrior. His story is told by the famous Sanskrit playwright, Kalidasa, in the epic, *Kumarasambhava*. Regular practice of this asana helps to develop your strength and endurance. The steps exercise your limbs and torso vigorously, reducing stiffness in your neck and shoulders. It also makes your knee and hip joints more flexible.

CAUTIONS
◆

Do not practise if you have a cardiac condition, palpitations, heartburn, diarrhoea, or dysentery. Women with menorrhagia and metrorrhagia should avoid this asana.

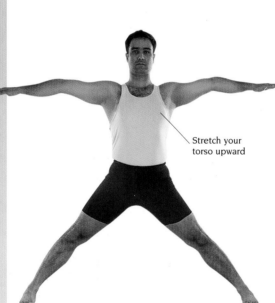

Stretch your torso upward

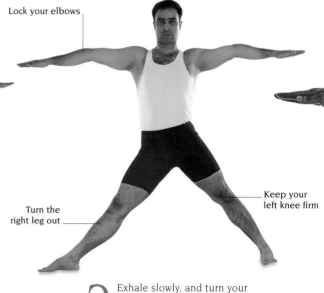

Lock your elbows

Keep your left knee firm

Turn the right leg out

1 Stand in Tadasana (*see page* 48) and inhale deeply. Jump, landing with your feet approximately 1.2m (4ft) apart. Your toes should point forward. Raise your arms out to the sides, in line with your shoulders (*see inset*). Your palms should face the floor and be in line with each other. Keep your fingers straight and stretched out. Press the little toe of each foot down on the floor. Consciously pull the inner sides of your legs up toward your waist.

2 Exhale slowly, and turn your right leg 90° to the right. Turn in your left foot slightly to the right. Ensure that your body weight is resting on your right heel and not on your toes. Keep your left leg stretched out and taut at the knee. To prevent this leg from slipping, make sure that your weight falls on the last two toes.

NOTE Focus on turning the right thigh out correctly. The thigh should turn at the same time – and to the same extent – as your right foot.

3 Exhale, and bend your right knee. Ensure that your right thigh is parallel to the floor. Keep the shin perpendicular to the floor, in line with your right heel. Pull the muscles of your right calf upward. Turn your head to the right. Stretch the arches and toes of both feet. Hold the pose for 30 seconds. Breathe evenly.

ADVANCED BEGINNERS Bend your right knee from the buttock bone and consciously push the flesh and skin of the thigh toward the knee. Stretch your arms out fully. Imagine they are being pulled apart in a tug-of-war.

BENEFITS

◆

Improves breathing capacity by expanding the chest

◆

Helps in the treatment of a prolapsed or slipped disc

◆

Alleviates the condition of a broken, fused, or deviated tailbone

◆

Reduces fat around the hips

◆

Relieves lower backache

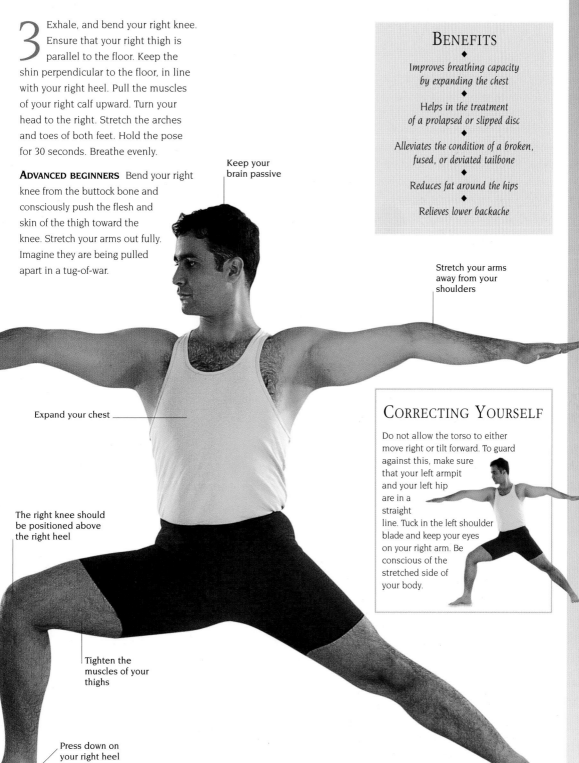

Keep your brain passive

Stretch your arms away from your shoulders

Expand your chest

The right knee should be positioned above the right heel

Tighten the muscles of your thighs

Press down on your right heel

CORRECTING YOURSELF

Do not allow the torso to either move right or tilt forward. To guard against this, make sure that your left armpit and your left hip are in a straight line. Tuck in the left shoulder blade and keep your eyes on your right arm. Be conscious of the stretched side of your body.

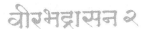

Virabhadrasana 2

ADVANCED WORK IN THE POSE

Do not bend your knee too rigidly and keep your bent leg relaxed. Consciously keep your brain passive. Your right buttock should be slightly lower than the right inner knee. Tighten your buttocks and broaden the hips. Press the outer edges of both your feet down on the floor. Feel the energy rise from the ankle to the knee. Push your chest out and expand your chest cavity to its full extent. Keep the left knee taut and lifted upward. If it drops, your chest will cave in. Maintain the stretch of your arms and shoulder blades away from your torso.

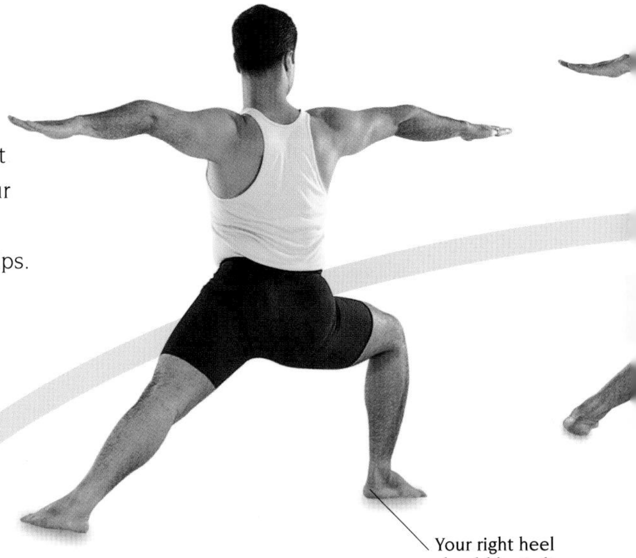

Your right heel should be in line with your right knee

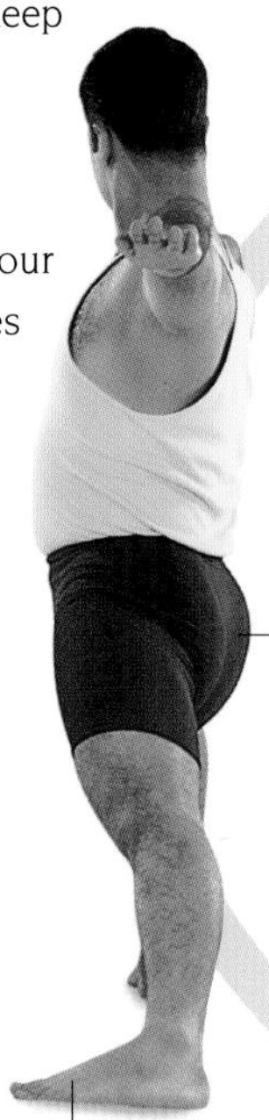

Keep your buttocks taut

Lock your elbows

Keep your toes separated and active

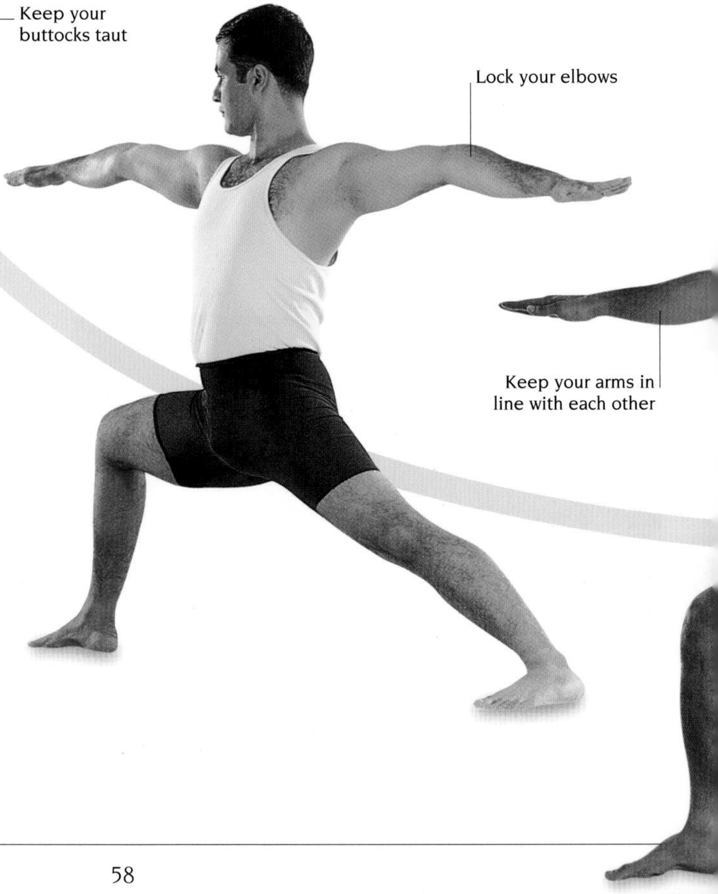

Keep your arms in line with each other

COMING OUT OF THE POSE

♦

Inhale, and straighten your right leg. Turn your feet, so that they face forward. Repeat this pose on the other side. Then exhale, and jump back to Tadasana.

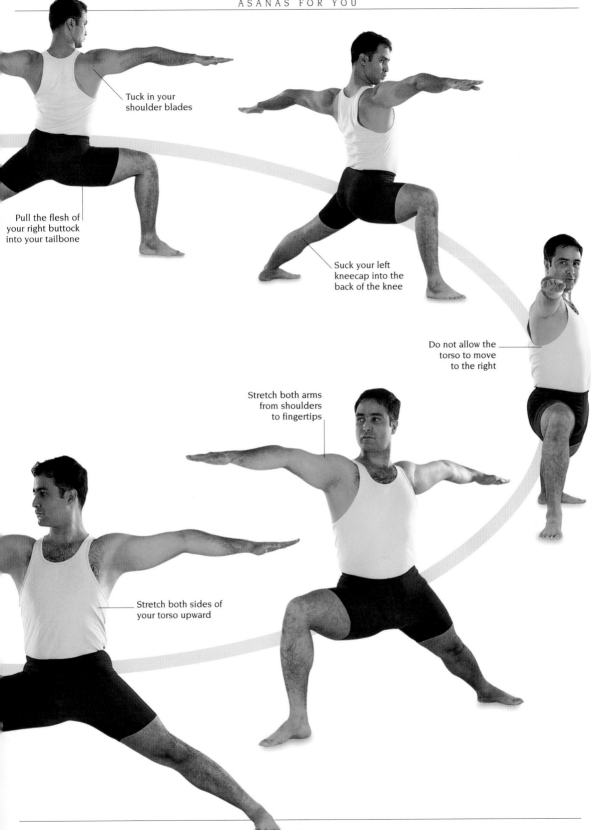

Tuck in your
shoulder blades

Pull the flesh of
your right buttock
into your tailbone

Suck your left
kneecap into the
back of the knee

Do not allow the
torso to move
to the right

Stretch both arms
from shoulders
to fingertips

Stretch both sides of
your torso upward

उत्थित पार्श्वकोणासन

Utthita Parsvakonasana

- Extended side stretch -

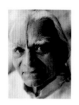

IN SANSKRIT, *utthita* means "stretch", *parsva* indicates "side" or "flank", while *kona* translates as "angle". In this asana, both sides of your body are stretched intensely, from the toes of one foot to the fingertips of the opposite hand. Remember to keep your body absolutely steady when practising this asana.

CAUTIONS
◆

If you have high blood pressure, avoid this asana. If you have cervical spondylosis, do not turn your neck or look up.

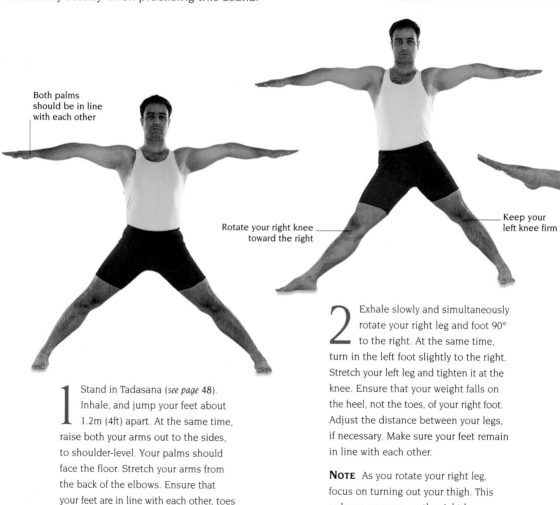

Both palms should be in line with each other

Rotate your right knee toward the right

Keep your left knee firm

1 Stand in Tadasana (*see page* 48). Inhale, and jump your feet about 1.2m (4ft) apart. At the same time, raise both your arms out to the sides, to shoulder-level. Your palms should face the floor. Stretch your arms from the back of the elbows. Ensure that your feet are in line with each other, toes pointing forward. Push down on the outer edges of your feet. Press the little toe of each foot down to the floor.

2 Exhale slowly and simultaneously rotate your right leg and foot 90° to the right. At the same time, turn in the left foot slightly to the right. Stretch your left leg and tighten it at the knee. Ensure that your weight falls on the heel, not the toes, of your right foot. Adjust the distance between your legs, if necessary. Make sure your feet remain in line with each other.

NOTE As you rotate your right leg, focus on turning out your thigh. This reduces pressure on the right knee.

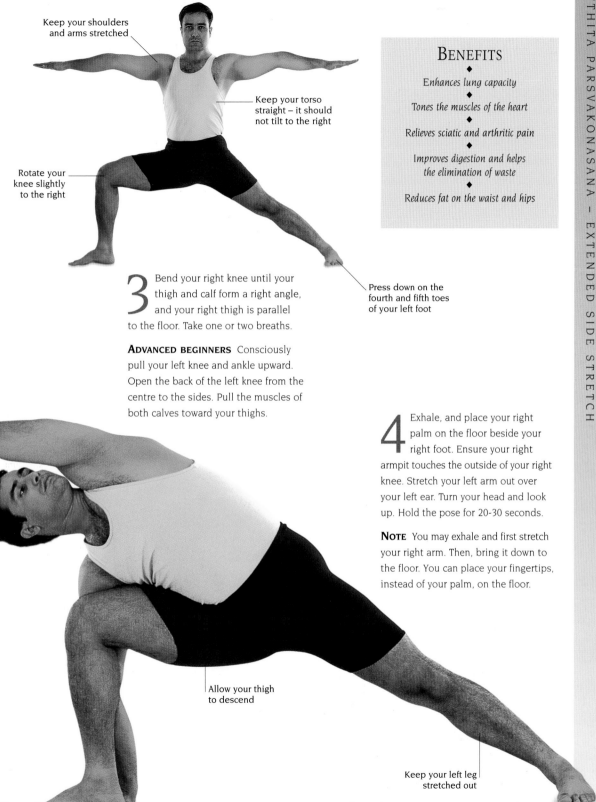

Keep your shoulders and arms stretched

Keep your torso straight – it should not tilt to the right

Rotate your knee slightly to the right

Press down on the fourth and fifth toes of your left foot

BENEFITS

◆

Enhances lung capacity

◆

Tones the muscles of the heart

◆

Relieves sciatic and arthritic pain

◆

Improves digestion and helps the elimination of waste

◆

Reduces fat on the waist and hips

3 Bend your right knee until your thigh and calf form a right angle, and your right thigh is parallel to the floor. Take one or two breaths.

ADVANCED BEGINNERS Consciously pull your left knee and ankle upward. Open the back of the left knee from the centre to the sides. Pull the muscles of both calves toward your thighs.

4 Exhale, and place your right palm on the floor beside your right foot. Ensure your right armpit touches the outside of your right knee. Stretch your left arm out over your left ear. Turn your head and look up. Hold the pose for 20-30 seconds.

NOTE You may exhale and first stretch your right arm. Then, bring it down to the floor. You can place your fingertips, instead of your palm, on the floor.

Allow your thigh to descend

Keep your left leg stretched out

उत्थित पार्श्वकोणासन

Utthita Parsvakonasana

ADVANCED WORK IN THE POSE

Your left arm is the "brain" of the pose (*see page* 45), so keep it stable and do not allow it to move. Increase the intensity of the stretch in this arm, pushing it away from the left armpit. Bring your lower shoulder blades into your back. Lift your left thigh slightly – this will help the right hand to descend more easily. Make sure you rest on the back of the right heel and do not allow dead weight to fall on your right thigh or palm. Keep your chest, hips, and left leg in line with each other. Stretch every part of your body, focusing especially on the spine. Feel a single, continuous stretch from your left ankle to your left wrist.

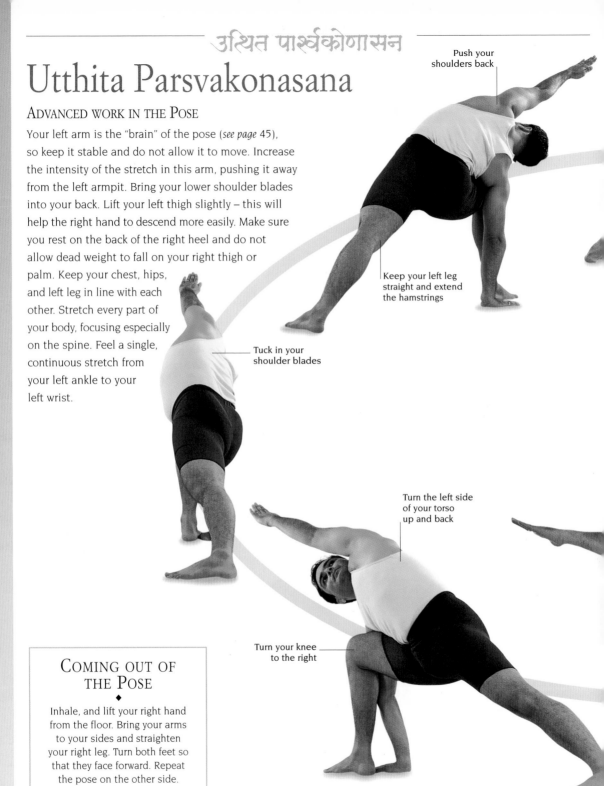

Push your shoulders back

Keep your left leg straight and extend the hamstrings

Tuck in your shoulder blades

Turn the left side of your torso up and back

Turn your knee to the right

COMING OUT OF THE POSE

◆

Inhale, and lift your right hand from the floor. Bring your arms to your sides and straighten your right leg. Turn both feet so that they face forward. Repeat the pose on the other side. Then exhale, and jump back to Tadasana.

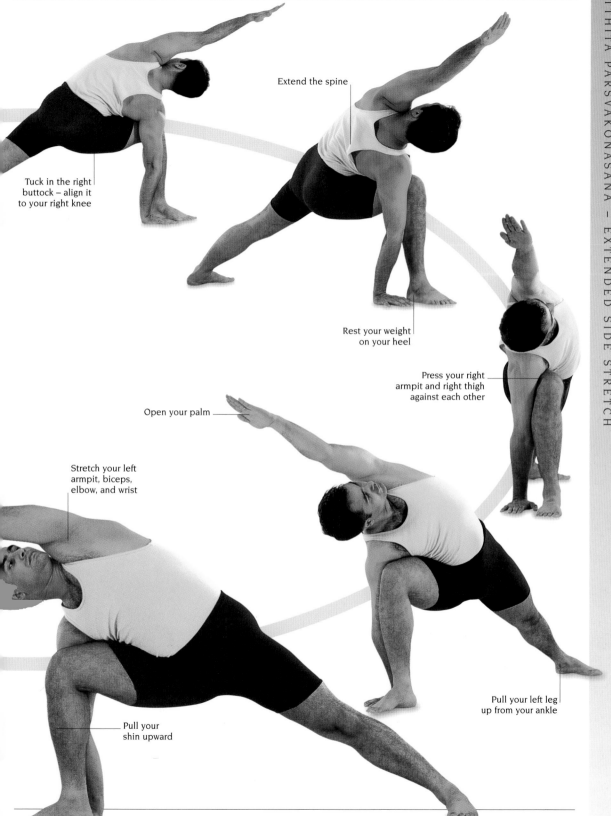

Tuck in the right buttock – align it to your right knee

Extend the spine

Rest your weight on your heel

Press your right armpit and right thigh against each other

Open your palm

Stretch your left armpit, biceps, elbow, and wrist

Pull your left leg up from your ankle

Pull your shin upward

पार्श्वोत्तानासन

Parsvottanasana

- Intense chest stretch -

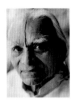

THIS ASANA GIVES an intense stretch to your chest. *Parsva* means "side" or "flank" in Sanskrit, while *uttana* indicates the great intensity of the final stretch. Regular practice of Parsvottanasana stimulates and tones the kidneys, an effect you can feel once you are comfortable in the final pose. The asana also helps to remove stiffness in the neck, shoulders, and elbows.

CAUTIONS
◆

If you have high blood pressure or a cardiac condition, omit Step 4. If you have dysentery or an abdominal hernia, practise this asana up to Step 4.

Push your shoulders back

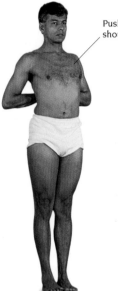

Press your wrists together

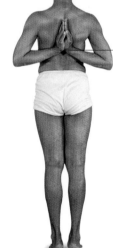

Ensure that your weight falls equally on both legs

1 Stand in Tadasana (*see page 48*). Loosen your arms by turning them inside and out several times. Join your fingertips together behind your back, with your fingers pointing down, toward your feet. Then rotate your wrists (*see inset*), until your fingers point to the ceiling.

NOTE If joining your palms is too difficult, take your arms behind your back, bend your elbows and rest each palm on the opposite elbow.

2 Move your joined palms up to the middle of your back. The little fingers of each hand should touch your back. Then, move your hands up your back (*see inset*) until they rest between your shoulder blades. Press your fingers together. Press your palms together by pushing your elbows inward. This will help to push your shoulders back and expand your chest even further.

3 Inhale and jump up, landing with your feet about 1.2m (4ft) apart. If your legs feel overstretched or uncomfortably close together, adjust the distance accordingly. When you feel that your body weight is distributed equally – and comfortably – on both legs, you have the distance right. Pause for a few seconds and exhale slowly.

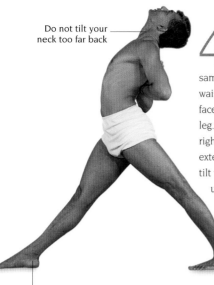

Do not tilt your neck too far back

Stretch your right foot so that it is completely extended

4 Inhale, and turn your right foot 90° to the right. Turn the left foot 75-80° to the right. At the same time, rotate to the right from the waist and hips. Ensure that your torso faces front and is in line with your right leg. Rest your weight on the heel of your right foot. Tighten your right knee and extend your chest, waist, and hips. Then, tilt your head and chest back and look up at the ceiling, making sure that you do not strain your throat. Press your palms to your back – do not allow them to slide down.

BENEFITS

◆

*Cools the brain
and soothes the nerves*

◆

*Relieves arthritis of the neck,
shoulders, elbows, and wrists*

◆

Strengthens the abdominal organs

◆

Improves digestion

◆

Tones the liver and spleen

◆

Reduces menstrual pain

Widen your elbows

Turn in your left kneecap slightly

Keep the right leg fully stretched

5 Exhale, extend the spine, and bend forward from the top of both your thighs. As you bend, lead with your sternum and do not allow your right knee to bend as you come forward. Take care to bend equally from both sides of the waist. Rest your chin on your right knee. Stay in the pose for 20-30 seconds. Breathe evenly.

NOTE If you find the final stretch difficult, then place your palms on the floor on either side of the right foot. Take care to stretch your back and neck gradually.

पार्श्वोत्तानासन

Parsvottanasana

ADVANCED WORK IN THE POSE

Maintain the stretch of your upper body, from the pelvis to the collar bones, while holding the pose. Elongate both sides of your waist evenly, to increase the stretch of your thighs. Bend down from your groin, keeping the perineum area passive. To ensure that your torso rests on the centre of your right thigh, move your abdomen slightly to the right, until your navel rests on the centre of your right thigh. Tighten the leg muscles and feel the stretch along the back of both legs. Push your spine down even further over your right leg. Move both your shoulders back, until both sides of your chest are equally expanded. Breathe evenly.

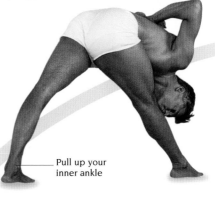

Pull up your inner ankle

Stretch your left leg

Keep your buttocks parallel to each other

Press the outer edge of your left foot to the floor

COMING OUT OF THE POSE
◆

Inhale, and lift your torso. Come back to a standing position, but do not raise your head immediately. Repeat the pose on the other side. Stretch out your arms to shoulder-level and jump your feet together. Stand in Tadasana.

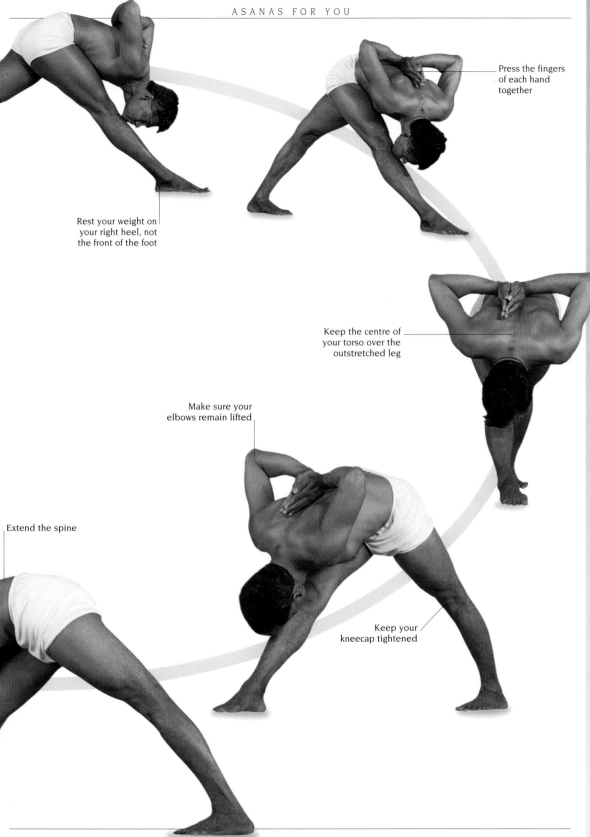

Press the fingers
of each hand
together

Rest your weight on
your right heel, not
the front of the foot

Keep the centre of
your torso over the
outstretched leg

Make sure your
elbows remain lifted

Extend the spine

Keep your
kneecap tightened

अधोमुख श्वानासन
Adhomukha Svanasana

- Downward-facing dog stretch -

IN THIS ASANA, your body takes the shape of a dog stretching itself. *Adhomukha* means to have your "face downward" in Sanskrit, and *svana* translates as "dog". The asana helps runners, as it reduces stiffness in the heels, and makes the legs strong and agile. Holding the pose for one minute restores energy when you are tired. This asana gently stimulates your nervous system, and regular practice will rejuvenate your whole body.

CAUTIONS
◆

If you have high blood pressure or frequent headaches, support your head with a bolster. If you are prone to dislocation of the shoulders, ensure that your arms do not rotate outward. Do not practise this asana in an advanced stage of pregnancy.

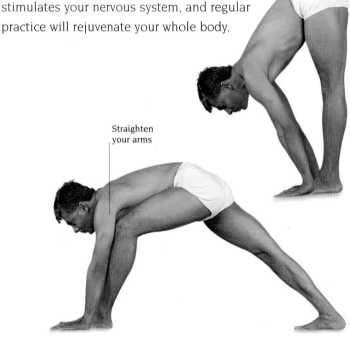

Straighten your arms

Keep your feet parallel to each other

Keep your arms fully stretched

1 Stand in Tadasana (*see page* 48). Exhale, and bend from the waist, placing each palm on the floor beside each foot.

NOTE If at first you cannot keep your legs straight, exhale and bend from your waist. Bend both knees and place your palms on the floor next to your feet.

2 Bend your knees and step back approximately 1.2m (4ft), one leg at a time. Keep your palms about 1m (3-4ft) apart. Make sure that the distance between your feet is the same as that between your palms.

3 Position your right leg in line with your right arm, and your left leg in line with your left arm. Stretch your fingers and toes. Raise your heels, tighten the muscles at the top of your thighs, and pull your kneecaps in. Then stretch the arches of your feet and bring your heels down to the floor again.

THE GURU'S ADVICE

"To make sure that my student's arms are straight, I stand on his hands to keep them firmly placed on the floor. Then I press his shoulder blades in, creating a right-angled triangle presentation of the pose. In this position, you should feel an intense stretch from your buttocks, along the dorsal and thoracic spine, right down to your palms."

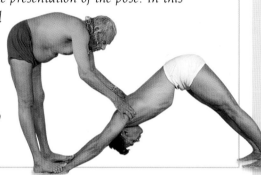

BENEFITS

Calms the brain and gently stimulates the nerves

Slows down the heartbeat

Reduces stiffness in the shoulder blades and arthritis in the shoulder joints

Strengthens the ankles and tones the legs

Relieves pain in the heels and softens calcaneal spurs

Checks heavy menstrual flow

Helps to prevent hot flushes during menopause

4 Pull your inner arms up from the elbows to the shoulders. Move your torso toward your legs. Feel the stretch from your palms to your heels. Now exhale, and stretching the base of your neck, lower the crown of your head to the floor. Hold the pose for 15-20 seconds.

ADVANCED BEGINNERS Before you lower your head, move the deltoids deep into the shoulder joints and lift your shoulder blades. Press both your palms down on the floor and pull your sternum up toward your diaphragm.

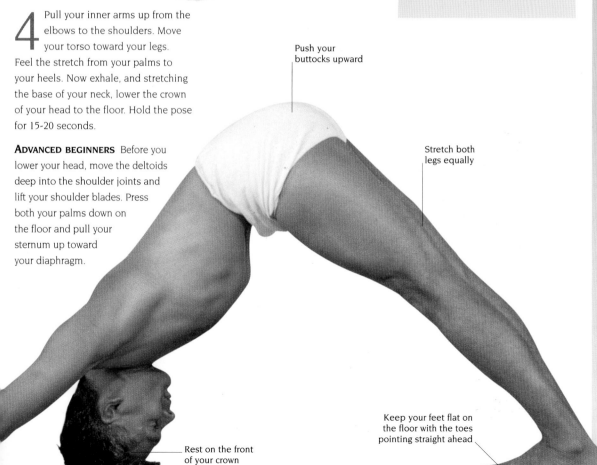

Push your buttocks upward

Stretch both legs equally

Rest on the front of your crown

Keep your feet flat on the floor with the toes pointing straight ahead

अधोमुख श्वानासन
Adhomukha Svanasana

ADVANCED WORK IN THE POSE

Move your legs as far back as possible. Ensure that both thighs are stretched equally – the inner and outer back edges should be parallel to each other. If your thighs are not parallel, they tend to shorten and lose their stretch. Similarly, keep your spine stretched out and do not compress it. Feel the energy in the spine flowing upward, from the neck to the buttocks, and not the other way round. Tuck in your shoulder blades and broaden your chest. As the chest opens out fully, your breathing becomes deep. Be aware of that depth.

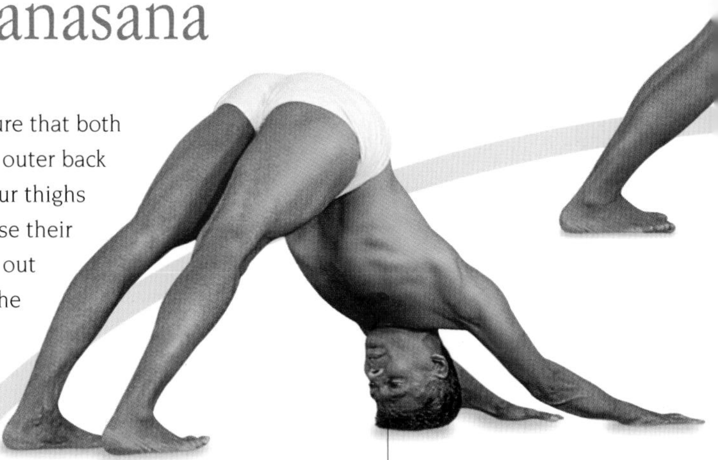

Rest on the front your crown

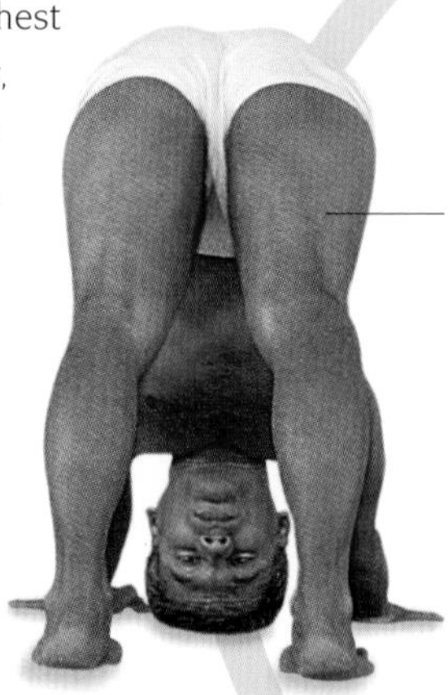

Keep your thighs parallel to each other

" The long an practice of asana. will brin

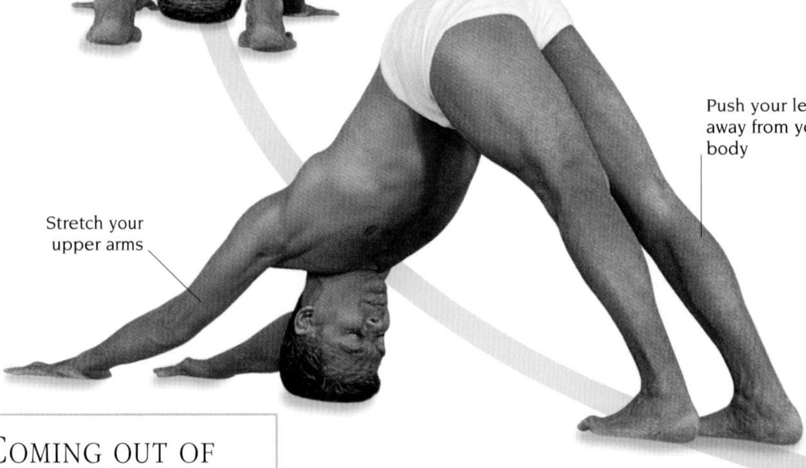

Push your legs away from your body

Stretch your upper arms

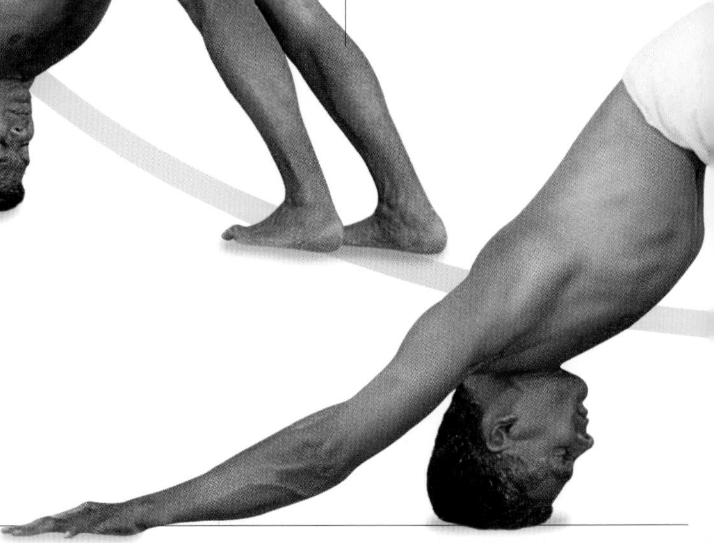

COMING OUT OF THE POSE

◆

Inhale, and gradually lift your head off the floor. Walk your feet toward your palms and come back to Tadasana.

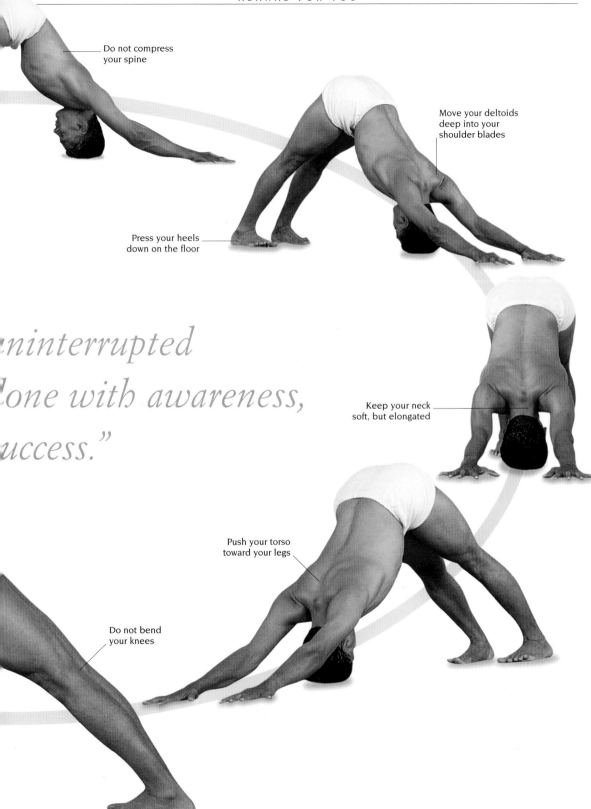

Do not compress your spine

Move your deltoids deep into your shoulder blades

Press your heels down on the floor

ninterrupted

one with awareness,

uccess."

Keep your neck soft, but elongated

Push your torso toward your legs

Do not bend your knees

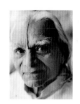

उत्तानासन
Uttanasana

- Intense forward stretch -

THE SPINE RECEIVES a deliberate and intense stretch in this asana. The word *ut* means "deliberate" or "intense" in Sanskrit, while *tana* connotes "stretch". The practice of Uttanasana helps the body and the brain recover from mental and physical exhaustion. This asana can help those who are prone to anxiety or depression as it rejuvenates the spinal nerves and brain cells. It also slows down the heartbeat.

CAUTIONS
◆

If you have a spinal disc disorder, stop at Step 3. Ensure that your spine is concave throughout the asana. Those prone to acidity or dizziness should practise this asana with the legs positioned slightly apart.

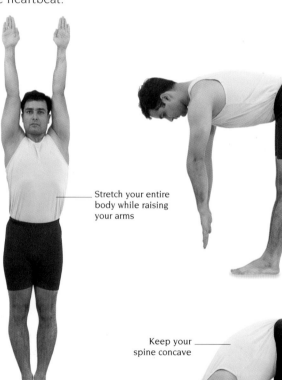

Stretch your entire body while raising your arms

Keep your spine concave

2 Exhale, and bend forward from the waist. Keep your legs fully stretched. Make sure that your body weight is placed equally on both feet. Extend your toes.

Extend your calf muscles

1 Stand in Tadasana (*see page* 48) with your legs straight and fully stretched. Tighten your kneecaps and then pull them upward. Raise your arms toward the ceiling, the palms facing forward. Stretch your whole body. Take one or two breaths.

3 Bend your torso further and place your palms on the floor in front of your feet. Separate your ankles a little, to free your lower back, buttocks, and legs. Consciously stretch the skin at the backs of your knees and thighs.

NOTE At first, lift your toes and press your heels down as you bend (*see inset*). Instead of your palms, you can rest your fingertips on the floor, until you are more flexible.

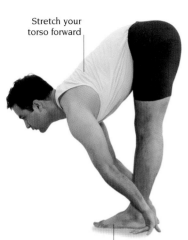

Stretch your
torso forward

Press the front of
your soles down
on the floor

4 Move your hands back and place them next to your heels. Rest on your fingers and thumbs, with the palms raised off the floor. Keep your thighs fully stretched – feel the energy flow along the back of your legs, into the waist, and down your spine. Pull your kneecaps into your knees, and keep both knees parallel to each other and fully opened out at the back. The pressure on the inner and outer edges of your feet should be equal.

CORRECTING YOURSELF

WRONG If your knees bend, the tailbone sticks out, impairing the pose.

RIGHT Stretch your thighs keeping the knee-caps locked and pushed upward.

Push your
hips forward

Extend your thighs
from the knees
to the hips

Stretch your arms
from your shoulders

5 Exhale, and push your torso closer to your legs until your face rests on the knees. Push your torso and abdomen further down toward the floor until your chin touches both knees. Your chin should not touch your chest, as this will cause your neck and throat to tighten, leading to pressure on the head. Hold the pose for 30-60 seconds, breathing evenly.

BENEFITS
◆
Relieves mental and physical exhaustion
◆
Slows down the heartbeat
◆
Tones the liver, spleen, and kidneys
◆
Relieves stomachache
◆
Reduces abdominal and back pain during menstruation

उत्तानासन

Uttanasana

ADVANCED WORK IN THE POSE

When you place your fingers on the floor, turn your arms out and stretch them downward. Imagine you are pushing the skin of your arms down from your armpits to your fingertips. Focus on your ribs. Consciously stretch each rib, from the bottom of your ribcage right up to your armpits. Then, descend even further from your armpits. This will open the back of your inner thighs. Feel a continuous stretch from your heels to the crown of your head.

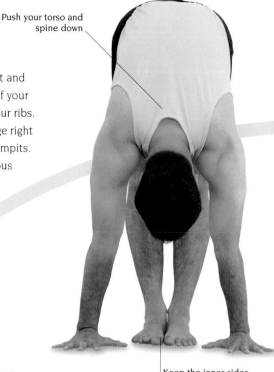

Push your torso and spine down

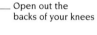

Open out the backs of your knees

Keep the inner sides of your ankles, knees, and thighs together

COMING OUT OF THE POSE

◆

Inhale, and raise your head without lifting your palms off the floor. Press your fingers into the floor and descend your armpits. Then, raise your torso gradually. Always be sure to come up with your back straight. Stand in Tadasana.

"Your body exist

your mind exists i

they come togethe

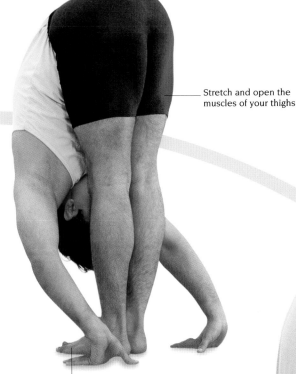

Stretch and open the muscles of your thighs

Keep your hips parallel to the floor

Extend your toes from the arches of your feet

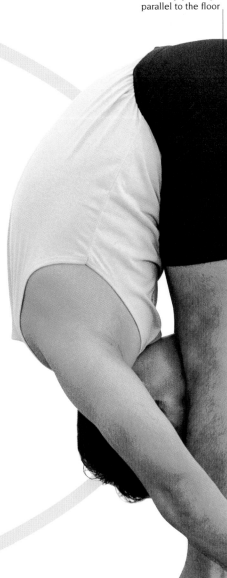

n the past and he future. In yoga, n the present."

वीरभद्रासन १

Virabhadrasana 1

- Warrior pose 1 -

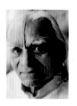

THIS ASANA, BASED ON a warrior pose, is a more intense version of Virabhadrasana 2 (*see page* 56). Both asanas are named after the mythic warrior-sage, Virabhadra. This vigorous asana strengthens your spine and increases the flexibility of your knees and thighs. The arms receive an intense stretch, and this expands the muscles of your chest and enhances the capacity of your lungs.

CAUTIONS
◆
Do not practise this asana if you have high blood pressure or a cardiac condition.

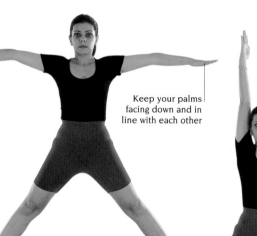

Keep your palms facing down and in line with each other

Lock your elbows

Pull up your pelvis

1 Stand in Tadasana (*see page* 48). Inhale and jump, landing with your feet about 1.2m (4ft) apart. Your feet should be in line, the toes pointing forward. Raise your arms up to shoulder-level, parallel to the floor. Lock your elbows. Press the little toes of both feet onto the floor. The outer edges of both feet should rest on the floor.

ADVANCED BEGINNERS For a more effective stretch, focus on the inner sides of your legs. Imagine that you are pulling the skin of both legs up from your heels to your waist.

2 Turn your wrists until your palms face the ceiling. Raise both arms until they are perpendicular to the floor and parallel to each other. Lift your shoulder blades and push them into your body (*see inset*).

ADVANCED BEGINNERS Your elbows are the "brain" of your arms (*see page* 45). Stretch from your elbows to your fingertips.

3 Exhale, and turn your torso and right leg 90° to the right. Then turn your left leg to the right. Rotate your torso from the chest as well as the waist. The more you rotate to the right and stretch your upper arms, the more effective the pose.

ADVANCED BEGINNERS Be conscious of your left leg, and concentrate on the stretch from the back of your heel to the back of your thigh.

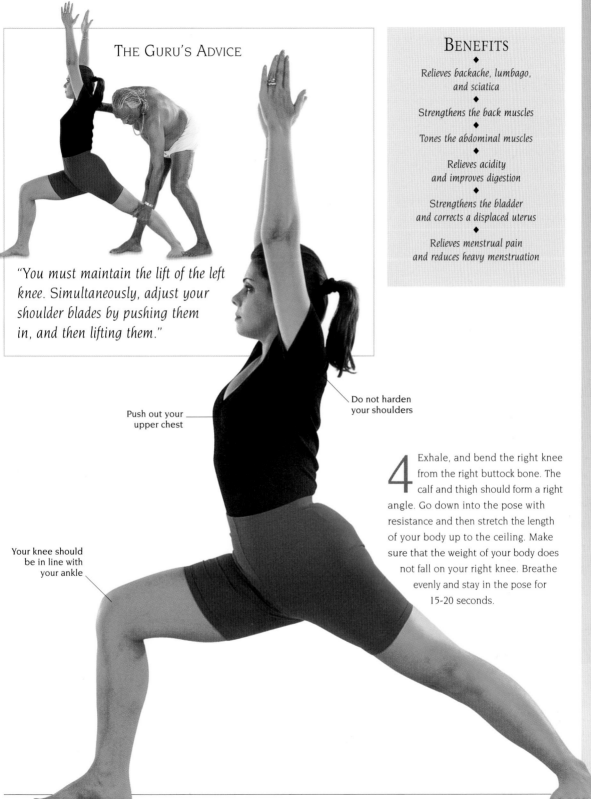

THE GURU'S ADVICE

"You must maintain the lift of the left knee. Simultaneously, adjust your shoulder blades by pushing them in, and then lifting them."

BENEFITS

◆

Relieves backache, lumbago, and sciatica

◆

Strengthens the back muscles

◆

Tones the abdominal muscles

◆

Relieves acidity and improves digestion

◆

Strengthens the bladder and corrects a displaced uterus

◆

Relieves menstrual pain and reduces heavy menstruation

Do not harden your shoulders

Push out your upper chest

Your knee should be in line with your ankle

4 Exhale, and bend the right knee from the right buttock bone. The calf and thigh should form a right angle. Go down into the pose with resistance and then stretch the length of your body up to the ceiling. Make sure that the weight of your body does not fall on your right knee. Breathe evenly and stay in the pose for 15-20 seconds.

वीरभद्रासन १

Virabhadrasana 1

ADVANCED WORK IN THE POSE

Feel the stretch in your back to experience the pose. Push your shoulder joints into the armpits, stretching your arms up higher. Ensure that the upper part of your body is symmetrical, with both armpits parallel to each other. Your face, chest, and right knee should be in line with your right foot. To avoid straining your right knee, turn your kneecap out toward the little toe of your right foot. Your weight should rest on the inner edge of your left buttock and on the outer heel of the left foot. Focus on your left side as it controls the harmony of the pose. Feel the energy flow up your left leg.

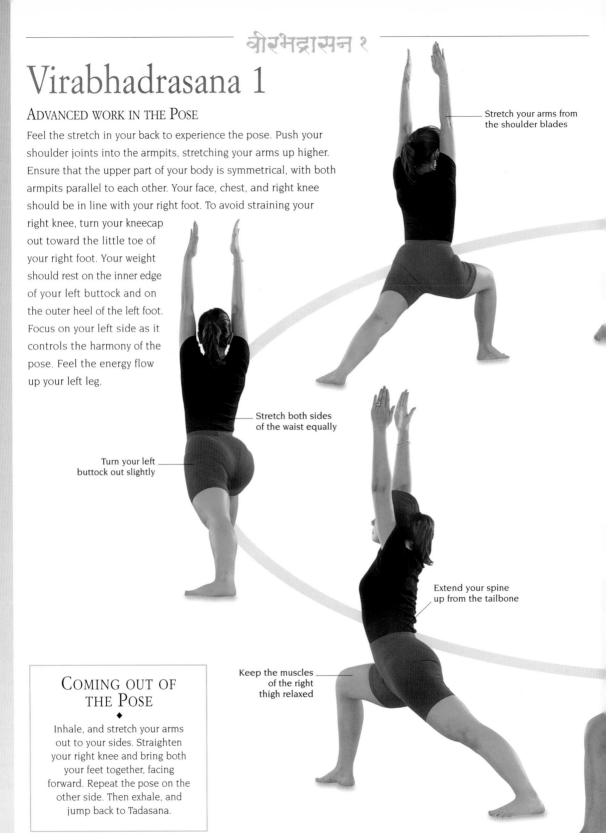

Stretch your arms from the shoulder blades

Stretch both sides of the waist equally

Turn your left buttock out slightly

Extend your spine up from the tailbone

Keep the muscles of the right thigh relaxed

COMING OUT OF THE POSE

◆

Inhale, and stretch your arms out to your sides. Straighten your right knee and bring both your feet together, facing forward. Repeat the pose on the other side. Then exhale, and jump back to Tadasana.

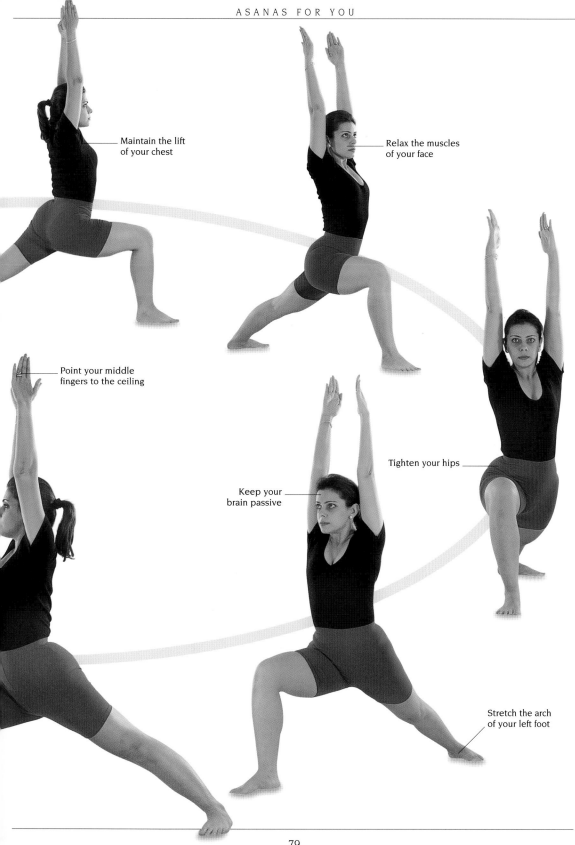

Maintain the lift
of your chest

Relax the muscles
of your face

Point your middle
fingers to the ceiling

Tighten your hips

Keep your
brain passive

Stretch the arch
of your left foot

Sitting Asanas

"Classic poses, when practised with discrimination and awareness, bring the body, mind, and consciousness into a single, harmonious whole."

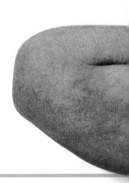

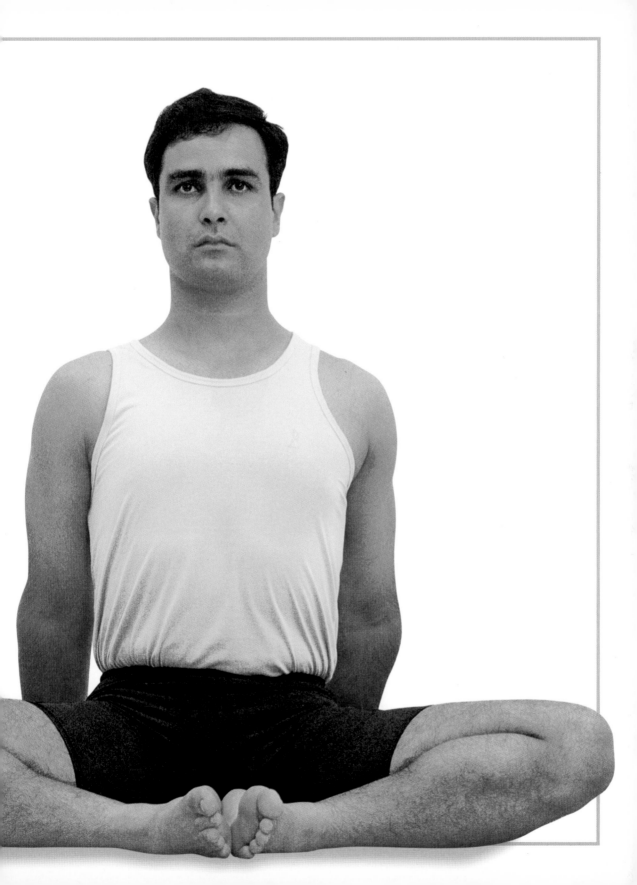

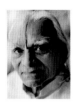

दंडासन

Dandasana

- Staff pose -

DANDASANA IS THE BASIC sitting pose for all forward bends. *Danda* means a "staff" or "walking stick" in Sanskrit, and regular practice of this asana improves your posture when seated. Your legs are rested during this asana, and it is recommended for people with arthritis or rheumatism of the knees and ankles. If you are prone to anxiety or mood swings, practising this asana helps to increase your will power and enhance your emotional stability.

CAUTIONS
◆

If your spine has a tendency to sag, or if you are experiencing a severe attack of asthma, practise this asana with the length of your spine supported against a wall.

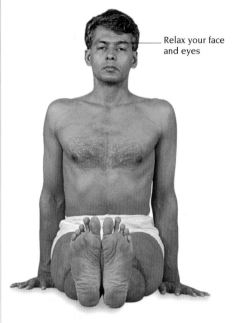

Relax your face and eyes

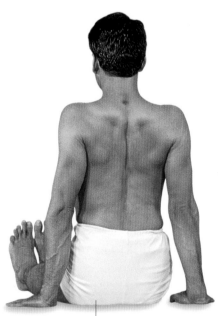

Rest on your buttock bones

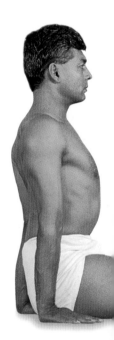

Spread out the soles of your feet

1 Sit on the floor with your legs stretched out. Move the flesh of each buttock out to the side with your hands (*see inset*), so that you are resting on the buttock bones. Keep your thighs, knees, ankles, and feet together. Place your palms on the floor beside your hips, with your fingers pointing forward. Lift your chest. Lock your elbows and straighten your arms.

BENEFITS

◆

Relieves breathlessness, choking,
and throat congestion in asthmatics

◆

Strengthens the muscles of the chest

◆

Tones the abdominal organs and lifts
sagging abdominal walls

◆

Reduces heartburn and flatulence

◆

Tones the spinal and leg muscles

◆

Lengthens the ligaments
of the legs

2 Tighten your quadriceps and pull
them toward your groin. Press
your thighs down on the floor,
and counter that pressure by lifting
your waist. Ensure that your diaphragm
is free of tension. Lift your ribcage and
keep your spine firm. Guard against
digging your lower spine into the floor.
Focus on keeping your head, neck, and
buttocks in a straight line. Hold the
pose for 20-30 seconds. Breathe evenly.

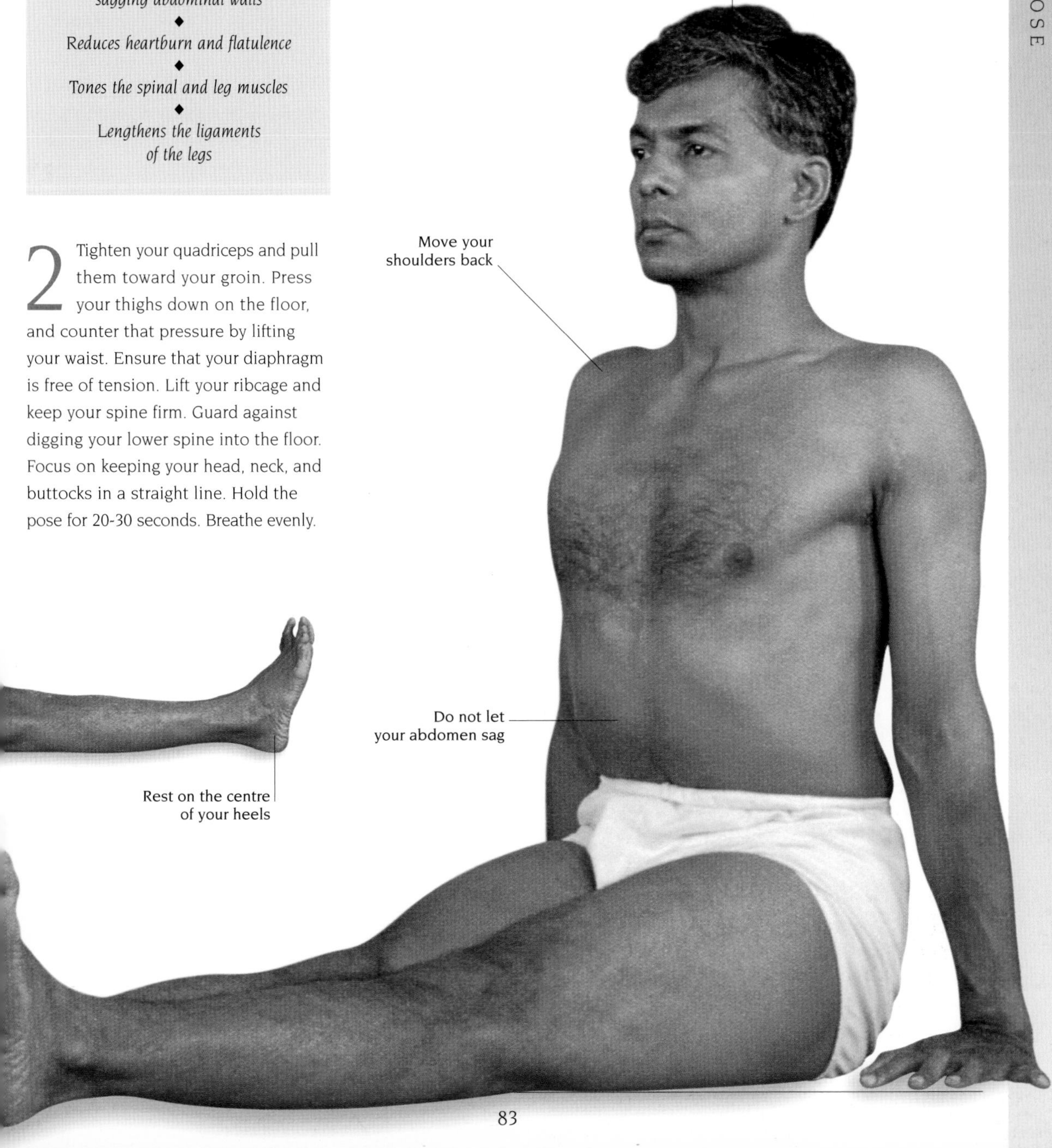

Keep your head
and neck erect

Move your
shoulders back

Do not let
your abdomen sag

Rest on the centre
of your heels

वीरासन

Virasana

- Hero pose -

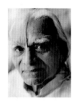

IN THIS ASANA, you assume the pose of a seated warrior. *Vira* in Sanskrit means "hero" or "warrior". Regular practice of this asana helps to develop your strength and endurance. The asana stretches the chest and increases your capacity for deep breathing. Virasana relieves stiffness in the joints and improves the flexibility of your whole body.

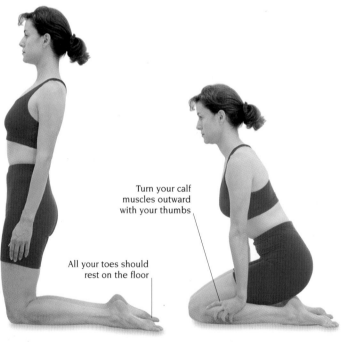

Turn your calf muscles outward with your thumbs

All your toes should rest on the floor

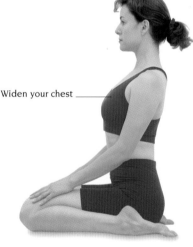

Widen your chest

1 Kneel on the floor with your knees together. Spread your feet about 0.5m (18in) apart, with your soles facing the ceiling.

ADVANCED BEGINNERS Adjust your ankles so that they stretch evenly from the arch to the toes and from the arch to the heels. Feel the energy flow smoothly in both directions.

2 Lean forward and rest your palms on your shins. Lower your buttocks toward the floor. Make sure that the inner side of each calf touches the outer side of each thigh. Turn your calf muscles outward and ensure that you turn your thigh muscles inward.

NOTE If you cannot rest your buttocks on the floor, place one sole on top of the other and rest your buttocks on them. Separate your feet.

3 Rest your buttocks on the floor. Do not sit on your feet. Place both palms on your thighs, close to the knees. Rest your weight on your thighs. Raise your waist and the sides of your torso, and press your shins firmly down on the floor.

Place your palms on your knees and push your thighs down. Lift your torso from the base of the pelvis.

ADVANCED BEGINNERS Imagine that your legs are tied to the floor, then lift your torso. Feel the energy flow upward from the bottom of your chest.

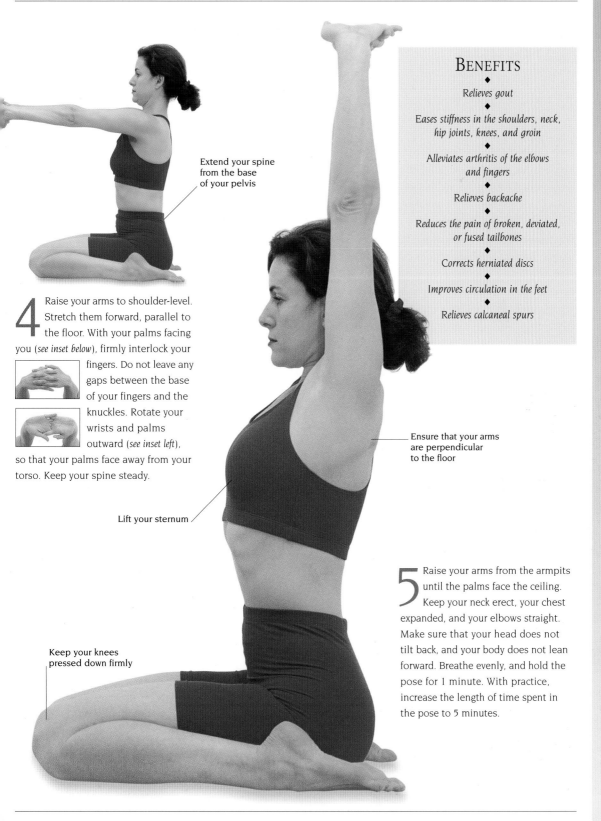

Extend your spine from the base of your pelvis

BENEFITS
◆

Relieves gout
◆
Eases stiffness in the shoulders, neck, hip joints, knees, and groin
◆
Alleviates arthritis of the elbows and fingers
◆
Relieves backache
◆
Reduces the pain of broken, deviated, or fused tailbones
◆
Corrects herniated discs
◆
Improves circulation in the feet
◆
Relieves calcaneal spurs

4 Raise your arms to shoulder-level. Stretch them forward, parallel to the floor. With your palms facing you (*see inset below*), firmly interlock your fingers. Do not leave any gaps between the base of your fingers and the knuckles. Rotate your wrists and palms outward (*see inset left*), so that your palms face away from your torso. Keep your spine steady.

Lift your sternum

Ensure that your arms are perpendicular to the floor

5 Raise your arms from the armpits until the palms face the ceiling. Keep your neck erect, your chest expanded, and your elbows straight. Make sure that your head does not tilt back, and your body does not lean forward. Breathe evenly, and hold the pose for 1 minute. With practice, increase the length of time spent in the pose to 5 minutes.

Keep your knees pressed down firmly

वीरासन

Virasana

ADVANCED WORK IN THE POSE

The intelligence of the body is energy, while the intelligence of the brain is consciousness. This energy moves with each action. When you stretch your arms upward, it is a physical action. Lifting the arms from the armpits after locking the elbows and deltoids, is an action done by the physiological body (*see page* 42). When you raise your arms, you will feel the energy move to the front of your legs. With every move, the energy in your legs flows to a different position. As the mind moves with this energy, focus on your legs. Imagine you are releasing the energy of your legs into the floor as you stretch your arms up even further. This will calm your mind and free your body of tension.

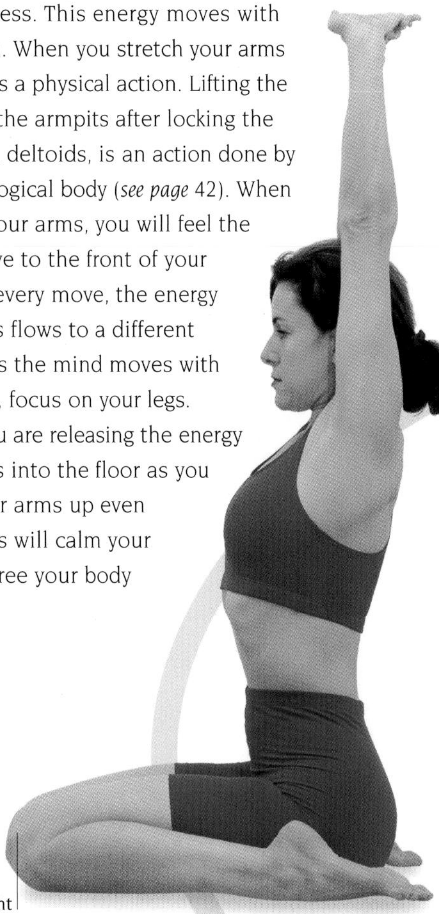

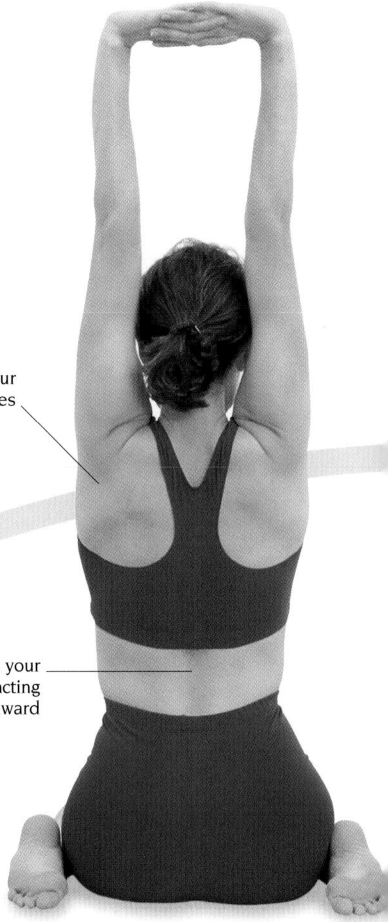

Tuck in your shoulder blades

Stretch and straighten your spine by sharply contracting the outer buttocks downward

Rest your weight on your knees

COMING OUT OF THE POSE

◆

Bring your arms down to your sides. Place your palms on the floor and raise your buttocks. Kneel, and then straighten your legs, one by one.

"The practic

change a person

a positiv

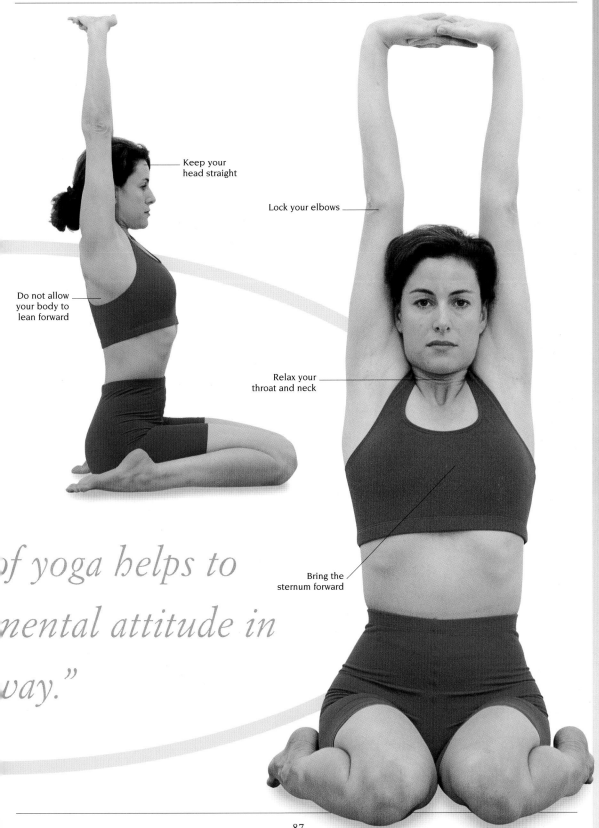

Keep your
head straight

Lock your elbows

Do not allow
your body to
lean forward

Relax your
throat and neck

Bring the
sternum forward

f yoga helps to

mental attitude in

vay."

बद्ध कोणासन

Baddhakonasana

- Fixed angle pose -

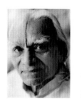

IN SANSKRIT, *baddha* means "bound" or "caught" and *kona* translates as "angle". Regular practice of Baddhakonasana increases the flow of blood to the abdomen, pelvis, and back. It helps to treat arthritis of the knee, hip, and pelvic joints. Pregnant women will experience less pain during labour and will be free of varicose veins if they hold the pose for a few minutes each day. You can practise this asana at any time, even just after a meal.

CAUTIONS
♦
Do not practise this asana if you have a displaced or prolapsed uterus.

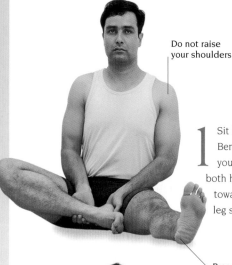

Do not raise your shoulders

Press your left heel down firmly

1 Sit in Dandasana (*see page* 82). Bend your right knee and hold your right ankle and heel with both hands. Draw your right foot toward your groin. Keep your left leg straight and resting on the floor.

2 Bend your left knee the same way as your right knee. Pull your left foot toward your groin, until the soles of both feet touch each other. Make sure that both heels touch the groin. Rest the outer edges of both feet on the floor.

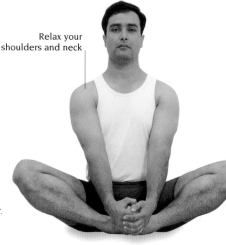

Relax your shoulders and neck

3 Hold your feet firmly near the toes with both hands. Pull your heels even closer to your groin. Stretch your spine upward. Widen your thighs and push your knees down toward the floor. Look straight ahead. Stay in this position for 30-60 seconds.

ADVANCED BEGINNERS Maintain your hold on your feet – the firmer your grip, the better the lift of the torso. Stretch out both sides of your chest.

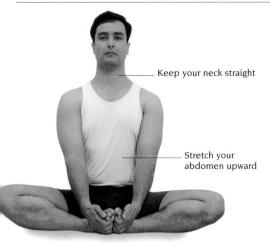

Keep your neck straight

Stretch your
abdomen upward

BENEFITS

♦

*Keeps the kidneys
and prostate gland healthy*

♦

*Helps to treat
urinary tract disorders*

♦

Reduces sciatic pain

♦

Prevents hernia

♦

*Relieves heaviness and pain in
the testicles, if practised regularly*

♦

Keeps the ovaries healthy

♦

Corrects irregular menstruation

♦

*Helps to open blocked fallopian tubes
and reduces vaginal irritation*

4 Push both your knees down by pressing your thighs firmly down on the floor. Stretch your knees away from the torso (*see inset*). This will also help to bring them down to the floor. Then, pull your heels back to the groin and relax your groin. Press your ankles and shins down to the floor and push your soles lightly toward each other. Straighten both your arms by stretching your torso upward even further. Breathe evenly.

NOTE It is difficult at first, to bring your knees down to the floor. Focus on your groin and consciously relax it.

5 Take your hands behind your back and place both palms on the floor. Keep your fingers pointing toward your buttocks. Push your shoulders back. Stay in this pose for 30-60 seconds, breathing deeply.

Ensure both sides of
your torso are parallel

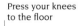

Press your knees
to the floor

बद्ध कोणासन

Baddhakonasana

ADVANCED WORK IN THE POSE

Once you are comfortable in the final pose, learn to
open your chest, stretching it outward from all sides.
Imagine that your legs are tied to the floor, so that
you raise your front ribs and lift your torso without
disturbing the position of your lower limbs. Then,
focus on your kidneys – imagine you are pulling them
into your body. Keep your back absolutely straight.
Inhale and exhale deeply, feeling your energy flow
from the bottom of your chest, over your shoulders
and down along the spine into the abdomen in one
continuous, cyclical flow. Gradually increase the
length of time you stay in this pose to 5 minutes.

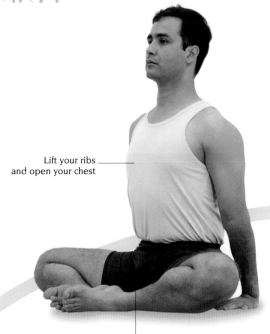

Lift your ribs
and open your chest

Keep your groin relaxed

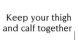

Keep your thigh
and calf together

" *All of us hav*

divinity in u

fanned int

COMING OUT OF
THE POSE
◆

Relax your arms and bring them
forward to rest on either side
of your body. Raise one knee
at a time, then straighten your
legs, one by one.
Return to Dandasana.

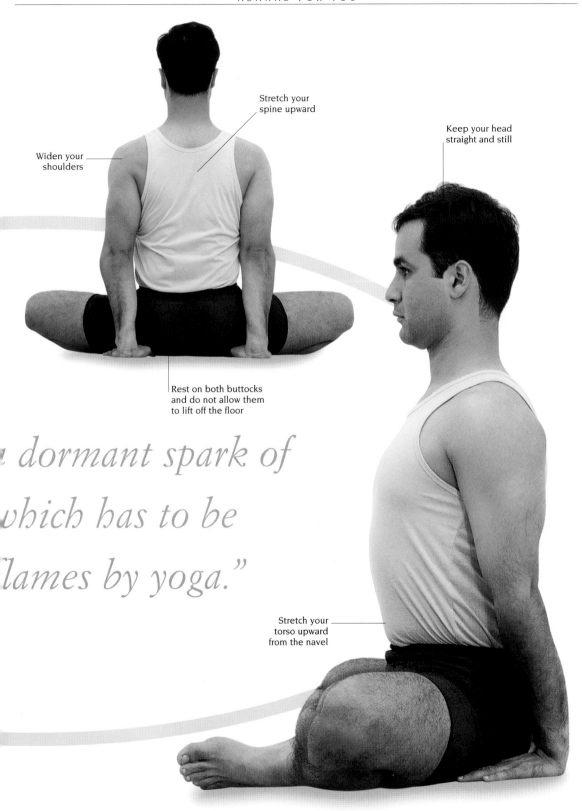

Stretch your
spine upward

Widen your
shoulders

Keep your head
straight and still

Rest on both buttocks
and do not allow them
to lift off the floor

dormant spark of

which has to be

flames by yoga."

Stretch your
torso upward
from the navel

Forward Bends

"Practise asanas by creating space in the muscles and skin, so that the fine network of the body fits into the asana."

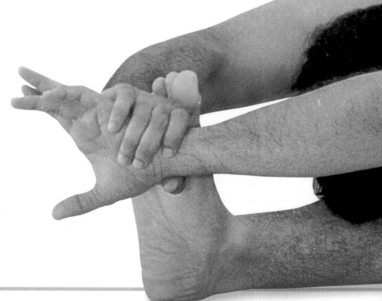

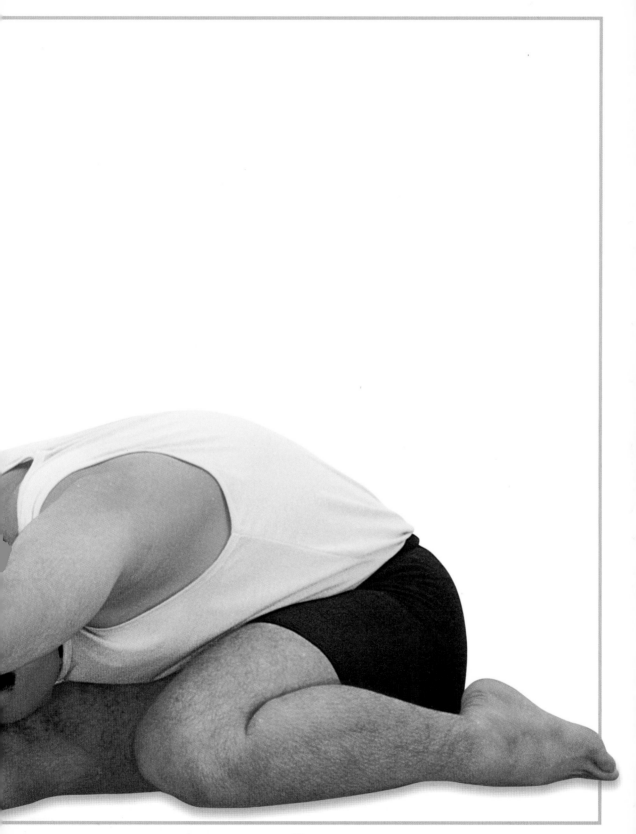

जानु शीर्षासन
Janu Sirsasana

- Head on knee pose -

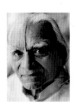

IN SANSKRIT, THE WORD for "knee" is *janu*, while "head" translates as *sirsa*. Practising this head-on-knee pose has a dynamic impact on the body and has many benefits. It stretches the front of the spine, eases stiffness in the muscles of the legs, and in the hip joints. It increases the flexibility of all the joints of the arms, from the shoulders to the knuckles. Forward bends like Janu Sirsasana rest the frontal brain and heart.

CAUTIONS
◆

To protect your hamstring muscles from damage, always open out the knee of the outstretched leg completely, extending it evenly on all sides. Do not allow the thigh of the same leg to lift off the floor.

1 Sit in Dandasana (*see page* 82). Bend your right knee and move it to the right. Pull your right foot toward your perineum until the big toe touches the inside of your left thigh. Make sure that your bent knee is pressed firmly down to the floor. Push back the bent knee until the angle between your legs is more than 90°. Keep your left leg straight. It should rest on the exact centre of the left calf.

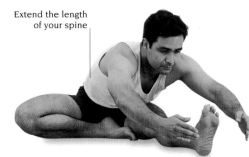

Extend the length of your spine

Stretch your arms from the armpits to the fingertips

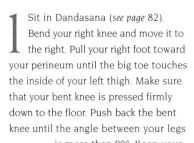

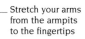

2 Stretch your left foot so that it feels as if the sole has widened, but keep your toes pointing straight up. Push the right knee even further away from your body. Then, lift your arms straight up above your head, with the palms facing each other. Stretch your torso up from the hips. Continue the stretch through your shoulders and arms.

3 Exhale, and bend forward from your hips, keeping the lower back flat. For a more effective stretch, push your torso down toward your waist to relax the spinal muscles. Stretch your arms toward your left foot and hold the toes.

NOTE If you cannot reach your toes, stretch as far along the leg as you can, holding on to your knee, shin, or ankle. Gradually, with practice, you will learn to stretch each part of your body separately – the buttocks, the back, the ribs, spine, armpits, elbows, and arms. Focus on keeping your left thigh, knee, and calf on the floor. Always press down on your thigh, not on your calf.

BENEFITS

◆

Eases the effects of stress on the heart and the mind

◆

Stabilizes blood pressure

◆

Gradually corrects curvature of the spine and rounded shoulders

◆

Eases stiffness in the shoulder, hip, elbow, wrist, and finger joints

◆

Tones the abdominal organs

◆

Relieves stiffness in the legs and strengthens the muscles of the legs

4 Now increase the stretch. Exhale and extend your arms beyond your left foot. Hold your right wrist with your left hand. Adjust your position – stretch the spine, press the right knee down to the floor. Keep your arms straight and lift your chest. Hold this position for 15 seconds, breathing evenly.

Keep your neck elongated and relaxed

Push your right knee further back

5 Exhale, and stretch your torso further toward the toes. Bring your forehead to your left knee, or as close to it as possible. Hold the pose for 30-60 seconds.

ADVANCED BEGINNERS Try to rest your nose on your knee, then your lips, and finally, rest your chin on your leg, just beyond the kneecap.

CORRECTING YOURSELF

When in the final pose, visualize the shape of your back. If it is rounded, as shown here, only a small part of the spine at the level of the shoulders is being stretched. Lengthen and flatten the lower spine and extend your arms out from your shoulder blades.

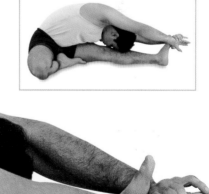

Push your torso toward your left foot

Rest the chest on your left thigh

जानु शीर्षासन

Janu Sirsasana

ADVANCED WORK IN THE POSE

When you are holding this pose, your sternum and abdomen should rest on the left thigh as though the leg and torso were one. One side of your back and torso might stretch more than the other – this is usually the same side as the outstretched leg. Be conscious of this, and try to equalize the stretch on both sides. Keep your elbows out, widening them to increase the expansion of your chest.

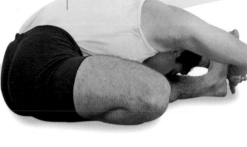

Do not allow the right side of your back to jut upward

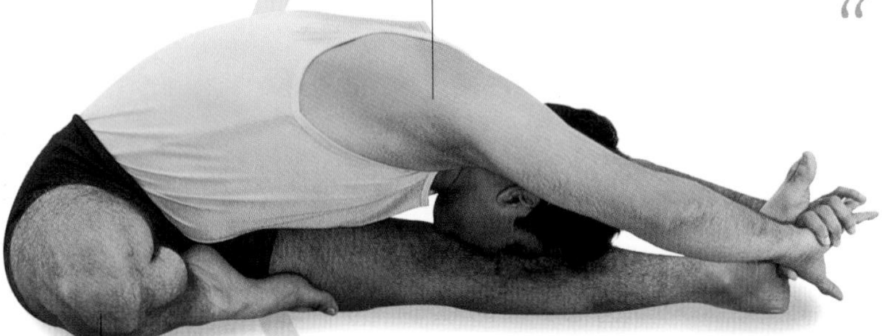

Stretch the arms from the armpits

Press your knee to the floor

"The intensit

increase an

momen

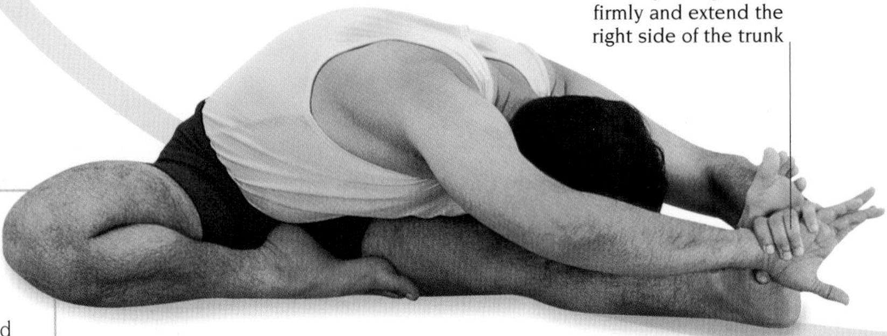

Hold your right wrist firmly and extend the right side of the trunk

COMING OUT OF THE POSE

◆

Inhale, then lift your head and torso slightly. After a few seconds, release your hands and sit up. Stretch out your right leg and sit in Dandasana. Now repeat the pose on the other side.

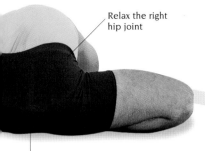

Relax the right
hip joint

Keep both buttocks
on the floor

Flatten and extend
the small of
the back

f the stretch should

ejuvenate from

o moment."

Keep your foot
pointed up – do
not allow it to tilt

Push your torso
toward the left foot

Relax the back of
the knee and keep
it on the floor

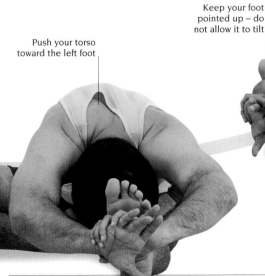

व्यंग मुखैकपाद पश्चिमोत्तानासन

Trianga Mukhaikapada Paschimottanasana

- Three parts of the body stretch -

IN SANSKRIT, the literal meaning of *trianga* is "three parts of the body". In this asana, the "three parts" comprise the buttocks, knees, and feet. The back of the body, which is known in Sanskrit as the *paschima* or "west", is stretched over *eka pada* or "one foot", and the *mukha* or "face" rests on the leg. Regular practice of this asana makes the whole body supple and agile.

1 Sit in Dandasana (*see page* 82). Bend your right leg back toward your right hip. Use your right hand to pull the ankle into place. Keep your left leg stretched out, making sure that it rests on the centre of your left calf and heel.

3 Raise your arms up toward the ceiling. Extend your torso upward, and feel the stretch from your waist to your fingertips.

NOTE To maintain your balance, keep the weight of your body on the bent knee. This will ensure that your torso does not tilt toward the left.

2 Keep your thighs together. Press your right knee down on the floor. The inner side of your right calf should touch the outer side of your right thigh. Balance equally on both buttocks. Make sure that your right buttock rests squarely on the floor (*see inset*). Rest your palms, fingers pointing forward, on the floor beside your hips.

Press the centre of the foot, ankle, and shin on the floor

Stretch the back of your left leg from thigh to heel

Straighten and stretch your toes

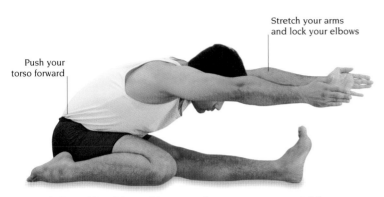

Push your
torso forward

Stretch your arms
and lock your elbows

BENEFITS
◆

*Tones and stimulates the
abdominal organs*
◆
*Assists digestion and counters
the effects of excess bile secretion*
◆
Reduces flatulence and constipation
◆
Creates flexibility in the knee joints
◆
*Corrects dropped arches
and flat feet*

4 Exhale, and bend forward from
the waist. Stretch both arms
beyond your left foot, with the
palms facing each other. Ensure your
thighs and knees are pressed together.
Rest on both buttocks – the essence of
the pose is getting this balance right.

ADVANCED BEGINNERS While you are
getting into the pose, the torso has a
tendency to tilt to the left. To guard against
this, shift your weight to your right side.
This will bring the centre of gravity to the
middle of your right thigh. Then, equalize
your weight on both buttocks.

5 Exhale, widen your elbows, and
push your torso toward your left
foot. Press both your wrists
against the sole of your left foot, then
hold your right wrist with your left hand.
First, touch your forehead to your left
knee, then place your nose and lips,
and finally, your chin, beyond your left
knee. Push your left buttock out and
rest on the inside of your left buttock
bone. Hold the pose for 30-60 seconds.

NOTE Stretch forward as far as you
can. With practice, you will learn to
hook your wrists around your foot.

Do not let your torso
tilt to the left

Extend your
shoulders and keep
your neck relaxed

त्र्यंग मुखैकपाद पश्चिमोत्तानासन

Trianga Mukhaikapada Paschimottanasana

ADVANCED WORK IN THE POSE

In the final stretch, make sure that your body weight is distributed evenly over your legs and buttocks. Keep your sternum in contact with your thighs. Both arms should be equally stretched forward. Make sure that the weight on the knee of the outstretched leg is equal to the weight borne by the bent knee. Focus on maintaining the centre of gravity of this pose at the middle of the right thigh. Extend the right side of your torso from the pelvic rim toward your head. Elongate the right side of your chest and waist, and expand the side of the ribs resting on your bent knee, so that your torso stretches further forward.

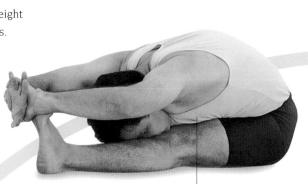

Rest your sternum on your thighs

Keep the muscles of your neck soft

" A yogi's brai
bottom of th
of h

Point your toes straight upward

COMING OUT OF THE POSE

◆

Inhale, raise your head and torso, and wait for a few seconds. Keep your back concave. Release your hands, then sit up and straighten your right leg. Repeat the pose on the other side.
Return to Dandasana.

Ensure that your bent knee remains pressed to the floor

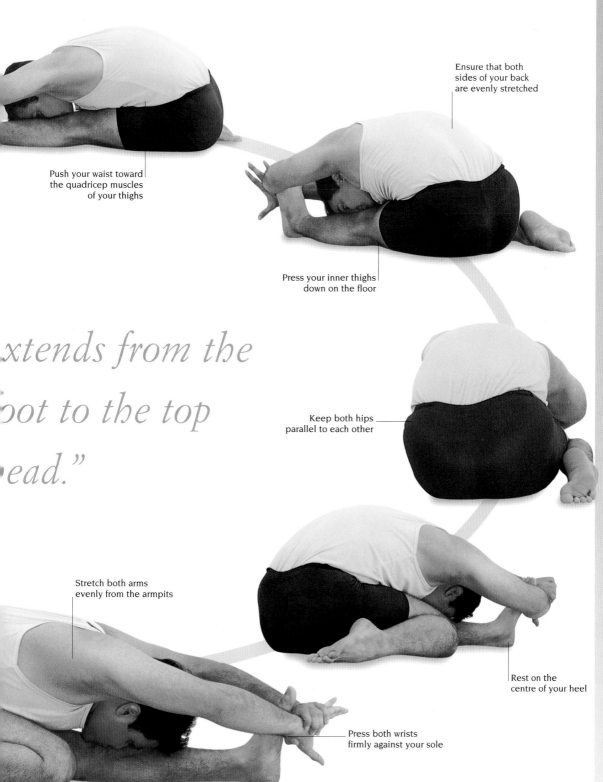

Ensure that both sides of your back are evenly stretched

Push your waist toward the quadricep muscles of your thighs

Press your inner thighs down on the floor

xtends from the

oot to the top

ead."

Keep both hips parallel to each other

Stretch both arms evenly from the armpits

Rest on the centre of your heel

Press both wrists firmly against your sole

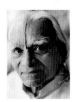

पश्चिमोत्तानासन
Paschimottanasana

- Intense back stretch -

T HE BACK OF YOUR BODY, from your heels to your head, is known as *paschim*, which means "west" in Sanskrit. Ut indicates "intense", while *tan* means "stretch". This asana stretches the length of your spine, allowing the life-force to flow to every part of your body. Resting your forehead on your knees, calms the active front brain, and keeps the meditative back brain quiet, yet alert.

CAUTIONS
◆

Do not practise this asana during, or just after, an asthmatic attack. Avoid this pose if you have diarrhoea. Do not allow your thighs to lift off the floor, as the muscles at the backs of your knees might rupture.

Keep your head straight

Stretch your legs out

1 Sit in Dandasana (*see page 82*). Keep your legs together. Stretch your heels, ensuring that both are evenly pressed down. Put your palms on the floor beside your hips. Take a few deep breaths. Now, stretch your arms above your head (*see inset*), with the palms facing each other. Stretch your spine upward.

2 Exhale, and stretch your arms toward your feet. Grip the big toe of your left foot with the thumb and first two fingers of your left hand. Do the same to your right toe with your right hand (*see inset*). Press your thighs down on the floor. The pressure on your thighs should be greater than that on your calves. This helps you stretch more effectively.

NOTE Focus on keeping your thighs flat on the floor. You must not allow them to lift off the floor. This is more important than holding your toes.

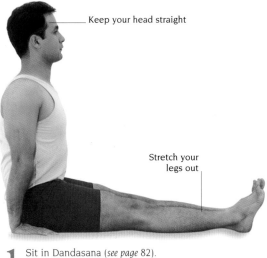

Hold your toes firmly

Do not raise the buttock bones off the floor

Press your shins and thighs firmly on the floor

BENEFITS

◆

Rests and massages the heart

◆

Soothes the adrenal glands

◆

Tones the kidneys, bladder, and pancreas

◆

Activates a sluggish liver, and improves the digestive system

◆

Helps to treat impotence

◆

Stimulates the ovaries, uterus, and the entire reproductive system

THE GURU'S ADVICE

"Stretch from the seat of the buttocks and feel the lightness in your buttocks. This is the heart of the perfect pose."

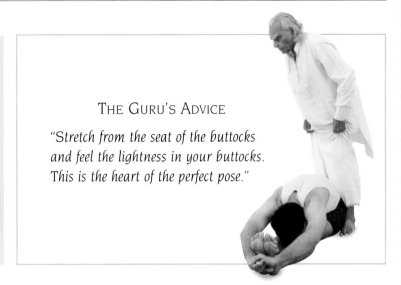

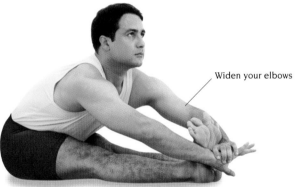

3 Make sure that you are sitting on your inner buttock bones and that your weight is distributed equally on them. Do not allow either buttock to rise off the floor. Then, hold your right wrist with your left hand.

ADVANCED BEGINNERS Hold the soles of your feet with the interlocked fingers of both hands. Breathe evenly.

Widen your elbows

4 Exhale, and lift your torso. Bend forward from your lower back, keeping your spine concave. Stretch forward from both sides of the waist. First, place your forehead firmly on your knees, and then push it toward your shins. Widen and lift your elbows. Do not allow them to rest on the floor. Hold the pose for 1 minute.

NOTE At first, rest your forehead on a folded blanket placed on your shins.

Stretch your arms from your shoulder blades

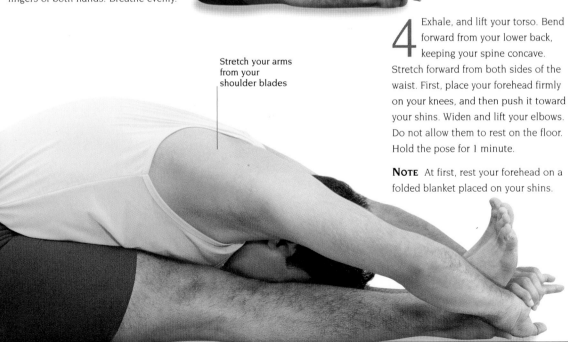

पश्चिमोत्तानासन

Paschimottanasana

ADVANCED WORK IN THE POSE

As you bend, keep your diaphragm as soft as dough. For a more effective stretch, bring your diaphragm closer to your chest as you lower your head. The front of your chest is the "brain" of this pose (*see page* 45). Bring it close to your thighs. Check that both sides of your chest are evenly stretched, so that there is a symmetry in the final pose. Press your forehead on your shins. Consciously descend your mind into the pose. Focus on your back – extend the skin of your back toward your head. Descend your spine completely. This will bring lightness and calm to the brain. Rejuvenate the stretch constantly. With practice, increase the duration of the pose to 5 minutes.

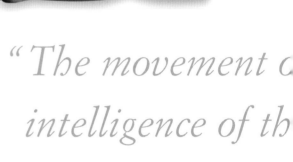

Keep the muscles of your neck passive

"The movement of intelligence of the and keep pac

Do not let your elbows move down

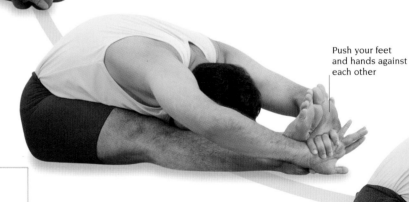

Push your feet and hands against each other

COMING OUT OF THE POSE
◆

Inhale, then raise your head and torso, keeping your back concave. Wait for a few seconds, then release your hands. Sit up and come back to Dandasana.

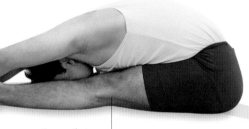

Keep your spine stretched

Ensure that your knees and thighs do not lift off the floor

Raise the inner sides of your upper arms

he body and the rain should synchronize with each other."

Compress your hips and keep them parallel to each other

Stretch forward from the base of your spine

Keep your armpits active and stretch them forward

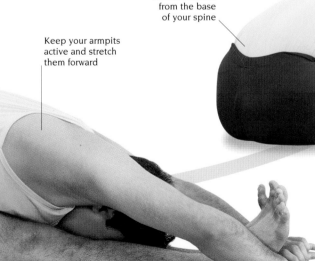

Rest on both buttocks equally

Twists

"If you practise yoga every day with perseverance, you will be able to face the turmoil of life with steadiness and maturity."

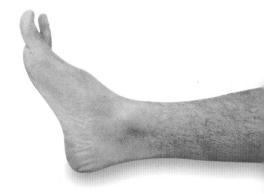

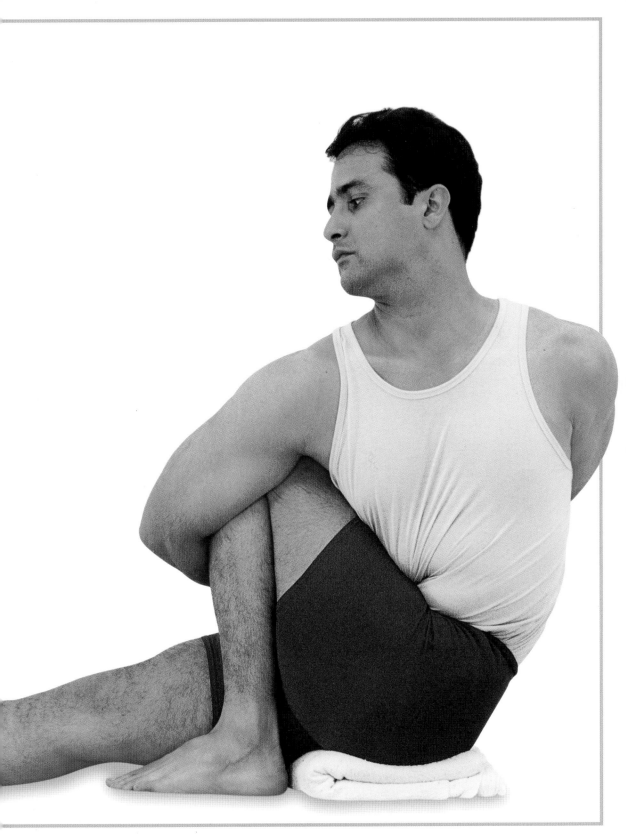

भरद्वाजासन
Bharadvajasana

- Torso stretch -

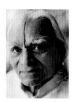

THIS ASANA IS NAMED after the ancient sage Bharadvaja, who was the father of the great warrior Dronacharya. Both are major characters in the Indian epic, *Mahabharata*. Regular practice of this asana teaches you to rotate your spinal column effectively, which increases the flexibility of your back and torso, and prepares you for the more advanced twists. It also massages, tones, and rejuvenates your abdominal organs.

1 Sit in Dandasana (*see page 82*). Place your palms flat on the floor behind your buttocks, with your fingers pointing forward. Bend your knees, and with your legs together, move your shins to the left. Make sure that your thighs and knees are facing forward. Breathe evenly.

Do not move your head

Take the left shoulder back

Keep your feet relaxed

2 Hold your ankles and bring your shins further to the left, until both feet are beside your left hip. The front of your left ankle should rest on the arch of your right foot (*see inset*). Extend the toes of your left foot and keep your right ankle pressed down to the floor. Rest your buttocks on the floor, not on your feet. Lift your torso, so that your spine is fully stretched upward. Pause for a few breaths.

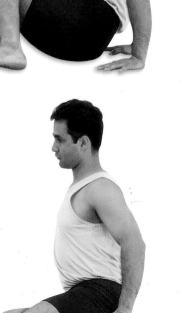

3 Exhale, then turn your chest and abdomen to the right, so that your left shoulder moves forward to the right, and your right shoulder moves back. Place your left palm on your right knee and rest your right palm on the floor. Revolve your right shoulder blade to the back and tuck in your left shoulder blade. Take one or two breaths.

BENEFITS

◆

*Relieves pain in the neck, shoulders,
and back*

◆

*Helps to keep the spine
and shoulders supple*

◆

*Eases a painful, stiff, sprained,
or fused lumbar spine*

◆

*Reduces discomfort
in the dorsal spine area*

◆

*Increases the flexibility of the back
and hips*

4 Press your right shin to the floor. This will help to lift your torso and turn it even further to the right. Rotate, until the left side of your body is in line with your right thigh. Turn your head and neck to the right. Inhale, and holding your breath, firmly press the fingertips of your right hand down on the floor. Then, exhale, and simultaneously raise and rotate your spine even more strongly to the right. Look over your right shoulder. Hold the pose for 30-60 seconds.

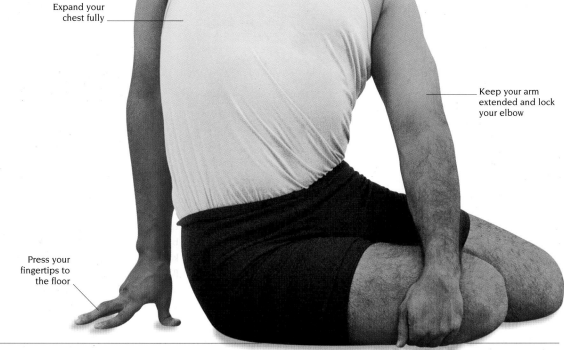

Turn your head
to the right

Expand your
chest fully

Keep your arm
extended and lock
your elbow

Press your
fingertips to
the floor

भरद्वाजासन

Bharadvajasana

ADVANCED WORK IN THE POSE

Once you have turned your neck and head to the right and rotated your torso, tuck in both your shoulders. Lift your sternum, keeping the spine erect as it turns on its axis. Do not change the position of your knees while turning, as they tend to move with the body. Ensure that your body does not lean back. Maintain the turn of your head and neck to the right. Keep the left hip and the left shoulder in line when you revolve your torso. Twist the spine strongly, turning it as far to the right as you can. Focus on the skin of your back. Try, consciously, to push your skin down from your neck, and pull the skin up from your lower back. Breathe evenly.

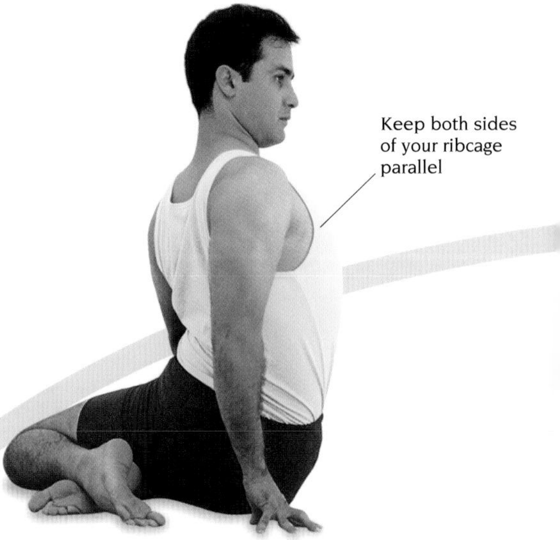

Keep both sides of your ribcage parallel

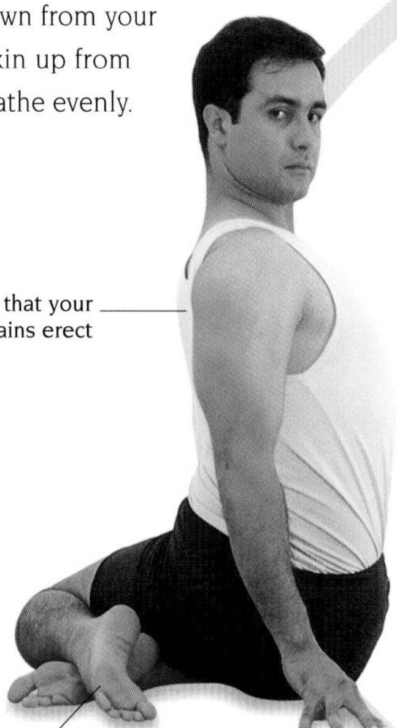

Ensure that your spine remains erect

Rest your left foot on the arch of the right foot

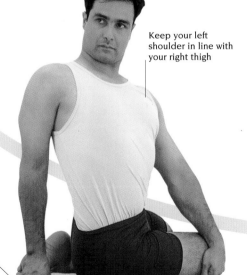

Keep your left shoulder in line with your right thigh

Press your fingers on the floor and lift the spine up

COMING OUT OF THE POSE

◆

Release your hands and bring your torso to the front. Straighten your legs. Repeat the pose on the other side. Come back to Dandasana.

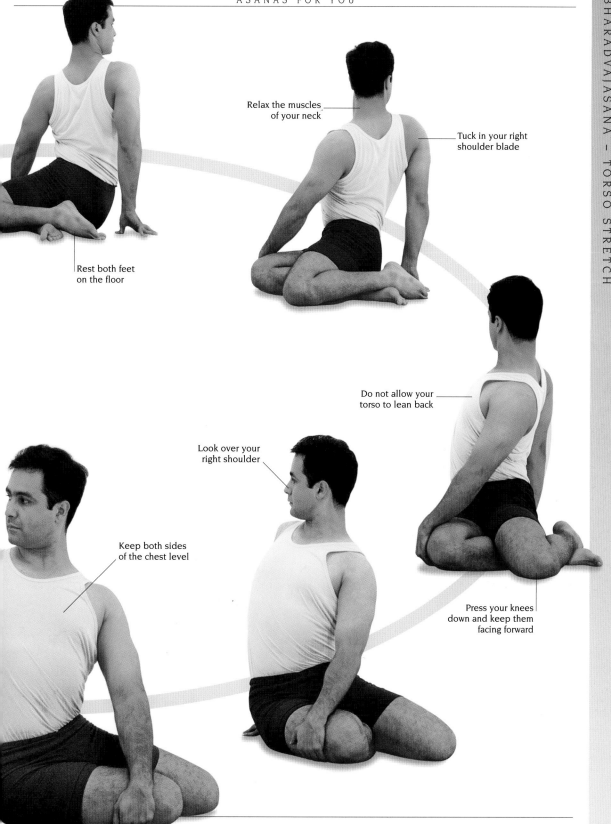

Rest both feet
on the floor

Relax the muscles
of your neck

Tuck in your right
shoulder blade

Do not allow your
torso to lean back

Look over your
right shoulder

Keep both sides
of the chest level

Press your knees
down and keep them
facing forward

मरीच्यासन
Marichyasana

- Torso and leg stretch -

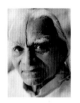

THIS ASANA IS DEDICATED to the sage, Marichi. His father was Brahma, creator of the universe, and his grandson was the sun god, Surya, the giver of life. Regular practice of the asana stretches your entire body and rejuvenates it. Marichyasana increases your levels of energy. The asana also massages and tones your abdominal organs.

CAUTIONS
◆

Do not practise this asana if you have diarrhoea or dysentery, or during a cold. Avoid this pose if you have a headache, migraine, insomnia, or when you are feeling fatigued. Do not practise during menstruation.

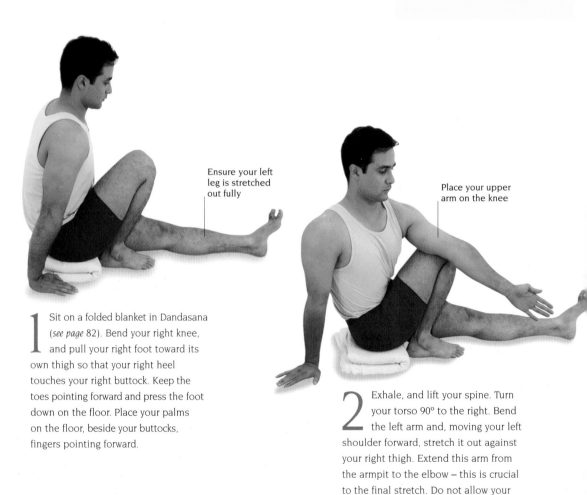

Ensure your left leg is stretched out fully

Place your upper arm on the knee

1 Sit on a folded blanket in Dandasana (*see page* 82). Bend your right knee, and pull your right foot toward its own thigh so that your right heel touches your right buttock. Keep the toes pointing forward and press the foot down on the floor. Place your palms on the floor, beside your buttocks, fingers pointing forward.

2 Exhale, and lift your spine. Turn your torso 90° to the right. Bend the left arm and, moving your left shoulder forward, stretch it out against your right thigh. Extend this arm from the armpit to the elbow – this is crucial to the final stretch. Do not allow your left leg to tilt to the left. Your weight should not fall on your right palm.

BENEFITS

◆

Increases energy levels

◆

Tones and massages the abdominal organs

◆

Improves the functioning of the liver, spleen, pancreas, kidneys, and intestines

◆

Reduces fat around the waistline

◆

Alleviates backache

◆

Relieves lumbago

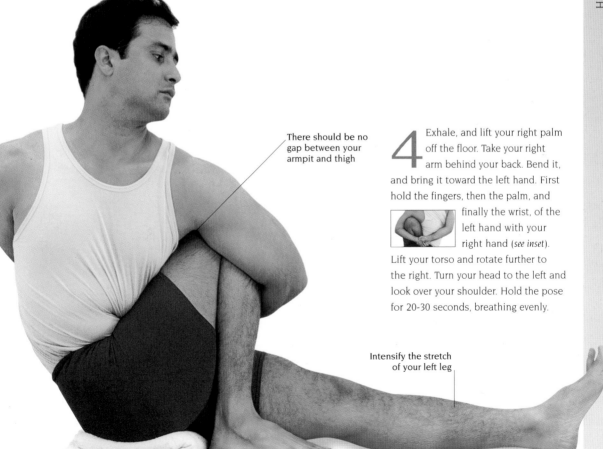

3 Press your right ankle down on the floor and turn your torso further to the right. Push your left armpit against the outer side of the right knee. This will help you rotate your torso more effectively. Ensure that you turn from your waist first, and then the chest. Exhale, and encircle your right knee with your left arm.

Press your right foot down on the floor

There should be no gap between your armpit and thigh

4 Exhale, and lift your right palm off the floor. Take your right arm behind your back. Bend it, and bring it toward the left hand. First hold the fingers, then the palm, and finally the wrist, of the left hand with your right hand (*see inset*). Lift your torso and rotate further to the right. Turn your head to the left and look over your shoulder. Hold the pose for 20-30 seconds, breathing evenly.

Intensify the stretch of your left leg

मरीच्यासन

Marichyasana

ADVANCED WORK IN THE POSE

This asana requires spinal action. Do not turn from your arms, but from your spine. The torso has a tendency to lean to the right in this pose, so consciously keep the left side of your body higher than the right. Stretch and lift the front of your spine. Bring your waist – and not just your chest – close to the middle of your right thigh. The entire length of the left side of your torso should be in contact with your right thigh. Bring your arms closer to each other and intensify your grip. The upper part of your right arm is the "brain" of the pose (see page 45), so keep it completely stable.

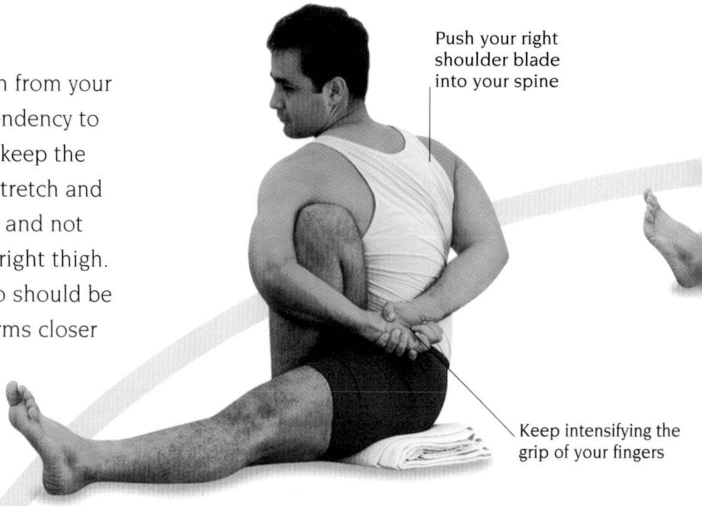

Push your right shoulder blade into your spine

Keep intensifying the grip of your fingers

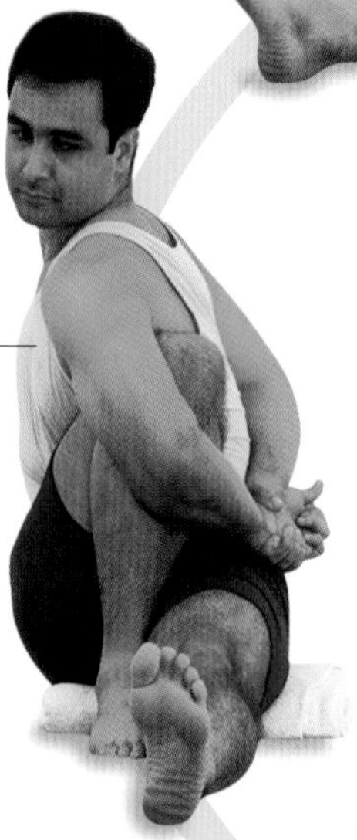

Move your whole body closer to the bent knee

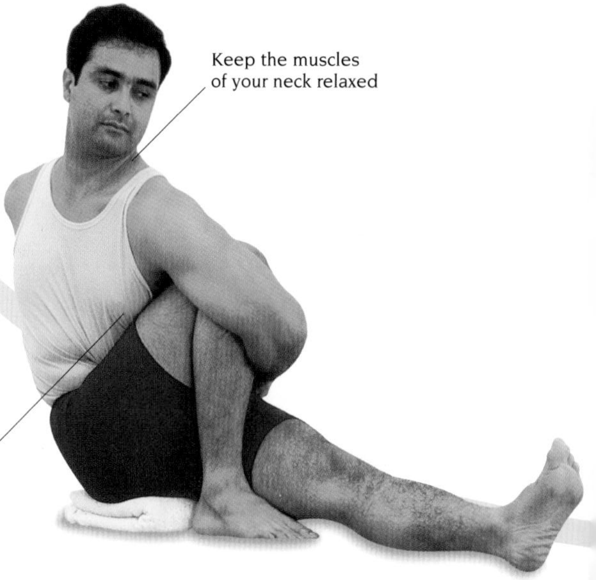

Keep the muscles of your neck relaxed

Your chest should touch the length of your right thigh

COMING OUT OF THE POSE
♦

Inhale, and holding your breath, rotate your spine to straighten it. Turn your head to face the front. Release your hands and straighten your leg. Repeat the pose on the other side. Return to Dandasana.

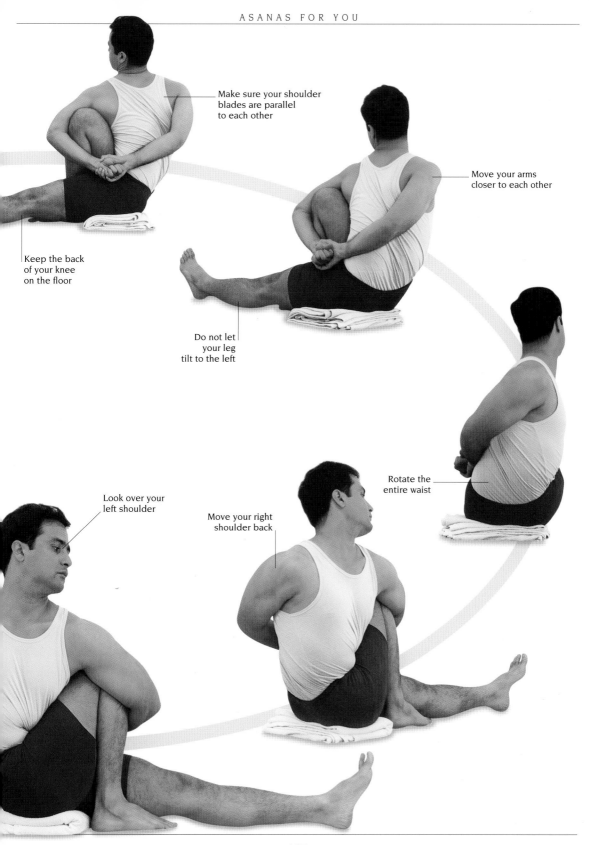

Make sure your shoulder blades are parallel to each other

Keep the back of your knee on the floor

Do not let your leg tilt to the left

Move your arms closer to each other

Rotate the entire waist

Look over your left shoulder

Move your right shoulder back

Inversions

"The practice of asanas purges the body of its impurities, bringing strength, firmness, calm, and clarity of mind."

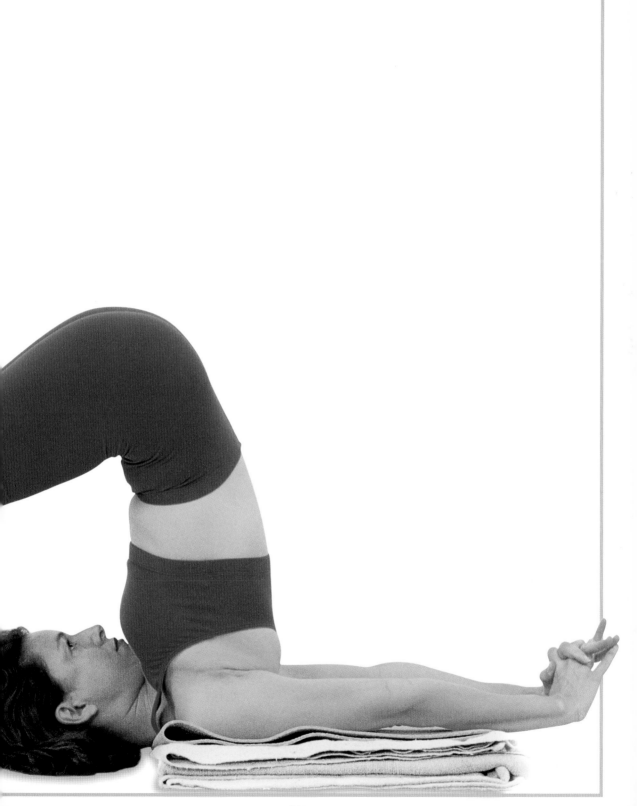

सालंब शीर्षासन

Salamba Sirsasana

- Headstand -

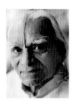

THE HEADSTAND IS ONE of the most important yogic asanas. The inversion in the final pose brings a rejuvenating supply of blood to the brain cells. Regular practice of this asana widens your spiritual horizons. It enhances clarity of thought, increases your concentration span, and sharpens memory. This asana helps those who get mentally exhausted easily. In Sanskrit, *sirsa* translates as "head", and *salamba* means "supported".

CAUTIONS
◆
Do not practise this asana if you have high blood pressure, cervical spondylosis, a cardiac condition, a backache, headache, or migraine. Do not start your yoga session with this pose if you have low blood pressure. Perform the asana only once in a session and do not repeat it – your body should not be overworked. Do not practise this asana during menstruation.

Firmly press your forearms on the floor and lift the shoulders upward

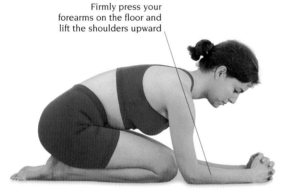

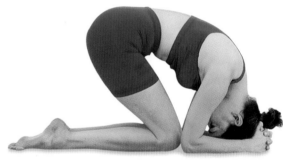

1 Kneel on the floor in Virasana (*see page* 84). Clasp the inside of your left elbow with your right hand and the inside of your right elbow with your left hand. Now lean forward and place your elbows on the floor. Ensure that the distance between your elbows is not wider than the breadth of the shoulders. Release your hands and interlock your fingers to form a cup with your hands (*see inset*). Keep your fingers firmly locked, but not rigid. Place your joined hands on the floor.

2 Place the crown of your head on the floor, so that the back of the head touches your cupped palms. Check that only the crown is resting on the floor, not the forehead, or the back of the head. In the final pose, your weight must rest exactly on the centre, not the back or front, otherwise, the pressure will fall on your neck or eyes, causing your spine to bend. Make sure that your little fingers touch the back of the head, but are not underneath it. Hold this position for a few seconds, breathing evenly.

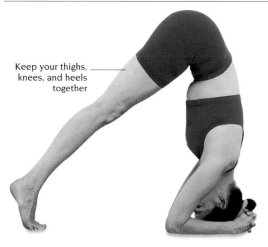

Keep your thighs, knees, and heels together

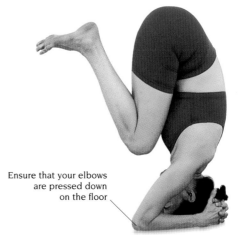

Ensure that your elbows are pressed down on the floor

3 Push up on the balls of your feet and straighten your knees. Keep your heels raised off the floor. To ensure that your torso is perpendicular to the floor, walk your feet toward your head, until the back of your body forms a vertical line from your head to the back of the waist.

4 Exhale, and bring your knees toward the chest. Press your toes down on the floor, and push your legs up, off the floor. This action resembles a hop, giving you the thrust to raise your legs. Bring your heels close to your buttocks.

NOTE If you find Steps 4–8 difficult, practise this asana against a wall (*see box below*).

SALAMBA SIRSASANA AGAINST A WALL

Practise against a wall, until you gain the confidence to practise without support. Place a folded blanket against the wall. Then follow Steps 1-3 (*see left and above*). Ensure that your cupped hands are placed not more than 5-8cm (2-3in) from the wall. If not, your weight will fall on your elbows, causing your spine to bend and your eyes to protrude. Follow Steps 4, 5, and 6 shown here. Initially, ask someone to help you raise your legs off the floor. To come out of the pose, follow the instructions on page 122 or reverse Steps 4-6.

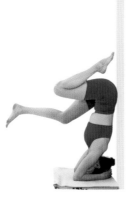

4 Once your torso is positioned perpendicular to the floor, rest your hips against the wall. Now bend your knees and raise your left foot off the floor with a swing. The swing should bring the thigh and knee to buttock level. Repeat the swing with the right leg.

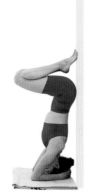

5 In this position, your hips and the balls of your feet rest against the wall. Adjust your body in the pose – press your elbows to the floor and stretch your upper arms. Follow the stretch through the armpits and along the torso to the waist.

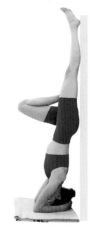

6 Straighten your legs, one by one, until your hips, legs, and heels rest against the wall. With practice, bring your hips away from the wall and let your head, arms, and torso bear your weight. Constant support of the wall will bend your spine.

सालंब शीर्षासन

Salamba Sirsasana

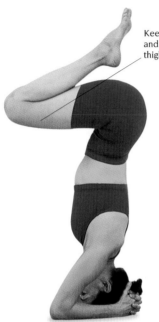

Keep your knees and the front of your thighs moving upward

Extend your toes

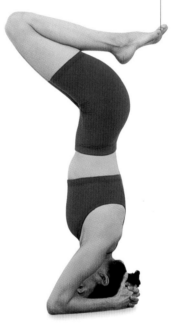

Point your knees toward the ceiling

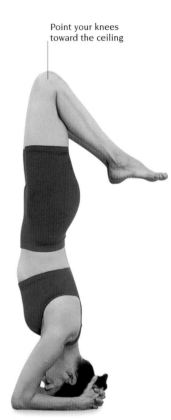

5 Press your elbows to the floor and lift your shoulders up, away from the floor (*see inset*). Exhale, and gently swing your knees upward in a smooth arc, until both your thighs are parallel to the floor. In this position, the entire upper body, from the head to the waist and hips, should be perpendicular to the floor. Do not move your elbows until you come out of the final pose.

6 Continue to move the knees upward, slowly bringing them to point to the ceiling. Keep the heels close to the buttocks. Focus on your balance and do not allow your torso to move during this action. Steps 5, 6, and 7 constitute a gentle, continuous movement, as you raise your legs toward the ceiling.

7 Once your knees are pointing to the ceiling, hold the pose for a few breaths. Make sure that the spine is straight. Tighten the buttocks. Ensure that your thighs are positioned perpendicular to the floor, your lower legs bent toward your back. Check that your shoulders do not tilt. Pause and get used to the feel of the position.

8 Straighten your knees to bring the lower legs in line with the thighs, so that your body forms a vertical line. Point your toes toward the ceiling. Tighten both knees, as in Tadasana (*see page* 48), and keep your thighs, knees, and toes together. The entire body should be balanced on the crown, not on the forearms and hands, which should simply support the balance in the pose. Stretch your upper arms, torso, and waist upward, along the legs to the toes, ensuring that your torso does not tilt. Steadiness and a constant lift of the shoulders ensure stability in the posture. Hold the pose for 5 minutes, breathing evenly.

Stretch the backs of your knees and thighs

Tighten the quadricep muscles

Expand your chest

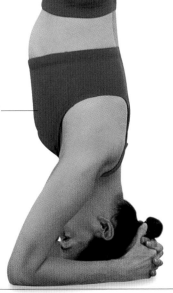

BENEFITS

◆

Builds stamina

◆

Alleviates insomnia

◆

Reduces the occurrence of heart palpitations

◆

Helps to cure halitosis

◆

Strengthens the lungs

◆

Improves the function of the pituitary and pineal glands

◆

Increases the haemoglobin content in the blood

◆

Relieves the symptoms of colds, coughs, and tonsillitis

◆

Brings relief from digestive and eliminatory problems, when practised in conjunction with Salamba Sarvangasana

CORRECTING YOURSELF

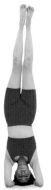 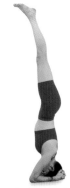

You may find that your legs lose alignment with the torso, either by wavering to the right or left. Check the position of your elbows and tighten your knees.

If you do not stretch the dorsal area and chest, your legs will swing forward and your buttocks jut back, When this happens, your weight falls on your elbows, not your head.

साल्ंब शीर्षासन

Salamba Sirsasana

ADVANCED WORK IN THE POSE

As you hold the pose, stretch your whole body, from the upper arms to the toes. Lift and widen the sternum so that your chest expands equally on all sides. Tighten your knees and bring your legs to the median plane. This will ensure that they are perpendicular to the floor. Pull the abdominal muscles in and toward the waist to extend the lower spine. You must practise this asana from the spine, not the brain. Balance is the key to this asana, not strength. You must develop the skill to balance effortlessly on the small surface area of the crown. This brings a feeling of lightness to the brain and complete relaxation to each part of the body.

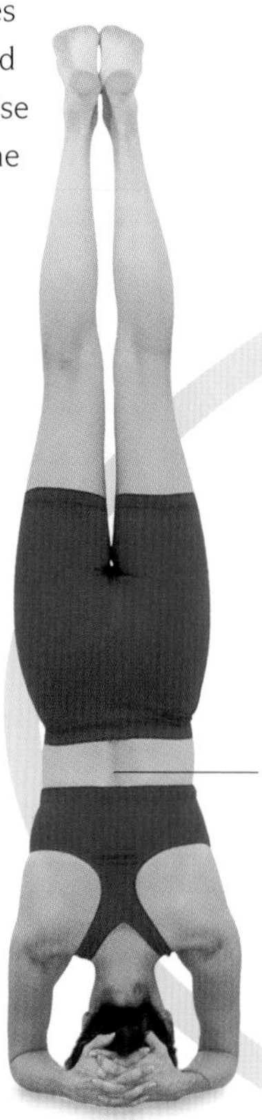

Extend the backs of the knees and stretch your shins

Stretch the biceps and deltoids up

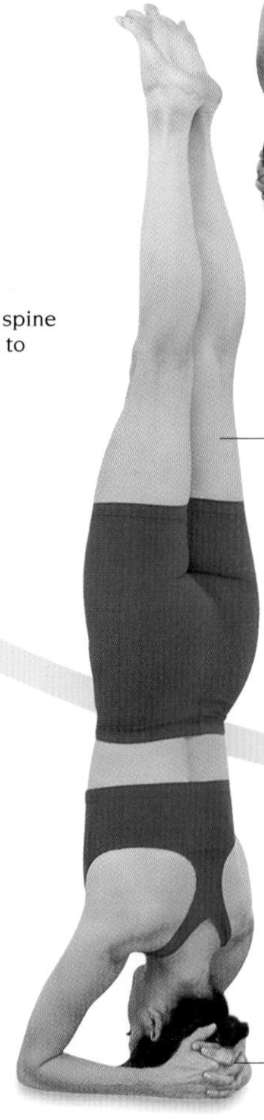

Lengthen the spine from the neck to the tailbone

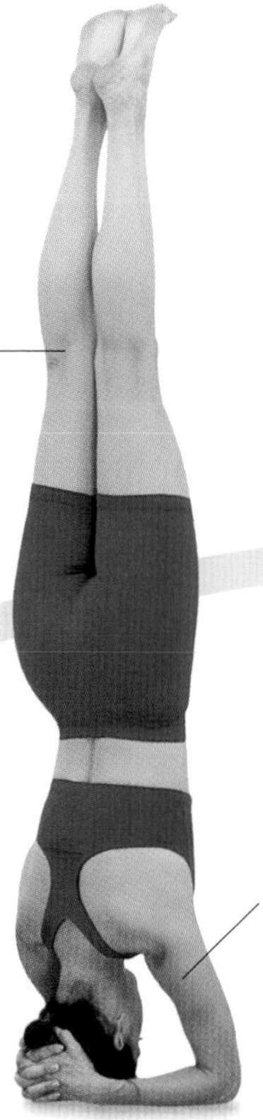

Elongate the inner sides of your legs

COMING OUT OF THE POSE
◆

Keep your legs straight and close together. Lower them until your toes rest on the floor. Bend the knees, kneel, and sit on your calves. Rest your forehead on the floor. Stay in this position for a few seconds before sitting up in Virasana.

Relax the fingers but keep them firmly locked

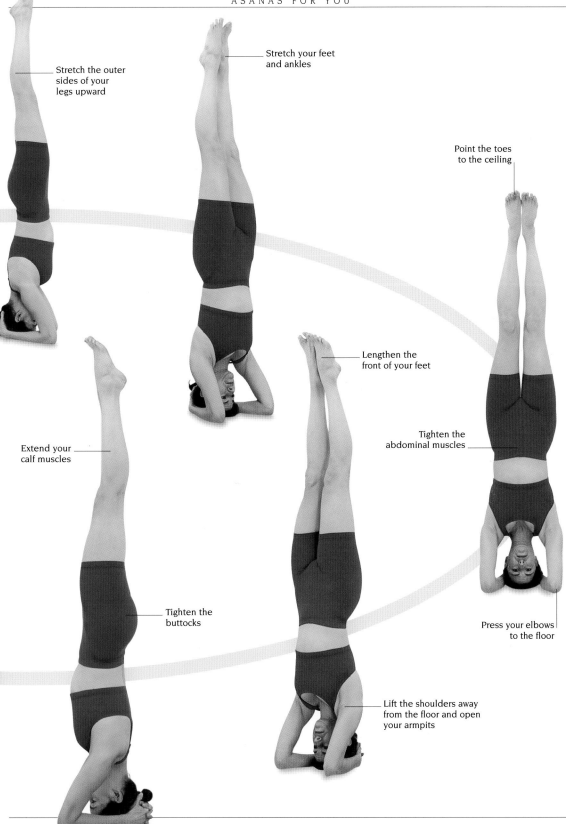

Stretch the outer sides of your legs upward

Stretch your feet and ankles

Point the toes to the ceiling

Lengthen the front of your feet

Extend your calf muscles

Tighten the abdominal muscles

Tighten the buttocks

Lift the shoulders away from the floor and open your armpits

Press your elbows to the floor

सालंब सर्वांगासन

Salamba Sarvangasana

- Shoulderstand -

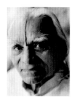

PRACTISING THIS ASANA integrates your mind with your body and soul. Your brain feels bright yet calm, your body feels light and infused with radiance. The inverted pose allows fresh, healthy blood to circulate around your neck and chest. This alleviates bronchial disorders and stimulates the thyroid and parathyroid glands. *Salamba* means "propped up" in Sanskrit, while *sarvanga* indicates "all the limbs" of the body.

CAUTIONS
◆

Do not practise this pose if you have diarrhoea, or during menstruation. People with high blood pressure should only attempt this asana immediately after holding the final pose of Halasana (*see page* 130) for at least 3 minutes.

Lift your sternum

Keep your toes, heels, and ankles together

Rest on the back of your head

1 Place a mat on 3 folded blankets, one on top of the other, on the floor. Lie down with your neck, shoulders, and back on the blankets. Rest your head on the floor. Stretch your legs and tighten your knees. Push the inner sides of your legs toward your heels. Press the outer sides of your shoulders down on the blankets. Raise your upper spine, but push your lower spine down on the blankets. Stretch your arms out close to your body, palms facing the ceiling. Make sure that your wrists touch your body. Raise and expand your sternum without moving your head.

2 Roll your shoulders back and pull in your shoulder blades. Turn your upper arms out slightly and stretch the inner sides of your arms toward the little fingers of each hand. Exhale, and bend your knees.

Relax the muscles of your face

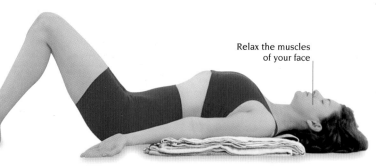

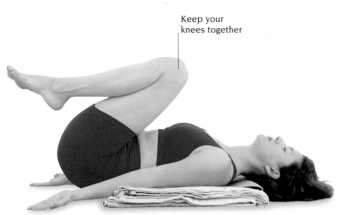

Keep your
knees together

BENEFITS

Alleviates hypertension

Relieves insomnia and soothes
the nerves

Improves the functioning of the thyroid
and parathyroid glands

Alleviates asthma, bronchitis,
and throat ailments

Relieves breathlessness and palpitations

Helps to treat colds and sinus blockages

Improves bowel movements
and relieves colitis

Helps to treat haemorrhoids

Alleviates urinary disorders

Helps to treat hernia

Helps to treat a prolapsed uterus and
reduces uterine fibroids

Relieves congestion and heaviness in the
ovaries, and helps to treat ovarian cysts

Reduces menstrual flow if practised
regularly between menstrual periods

3 Without moving the upper part of your body, exhale and raise your hips and buttocks off the floor. Bring your knees over your chest.

NOTE If you find it difficult, at first, to raise your hips off the floor, ask a helper to hold your ankles and push your bent legs toward your head. At the same time, lift your hips and back off the floor and come to the final pose. Keep your body firm, and rest your back against your helper's knees. Alternatively, once you have been helped to raise your legs off the floor, follow Steps 5, 6, and 7 on the next page.

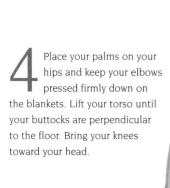

Tighten your
buttocks

Keep your shins
pressed together

4 Place your palms on your hips and keep your elbows pressed firmly down on the blankets. Lift your torso until your buttocks are perpendicular to the floor. Bring your knees toward your head.

SALAMBA SARVANGASANA – SHOULDERSTAND

सालंब सर्वांगासन

Salamba Sarvangasana

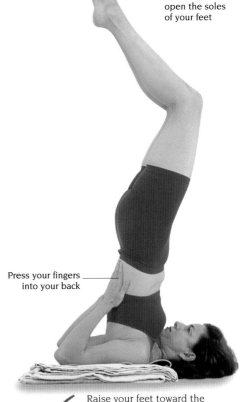

5 Now, slide your hands down to the middle of your back, so that your palms cover your kidneys (*see inset*). Point your thumbs toward the front of your body and your fingers toward the spine. Exhale, and raise your torso, hips, and knees, until your chest touches your chin. Breathe evenly.

Stretch and open the soles of your feet

Press your fingers into your back

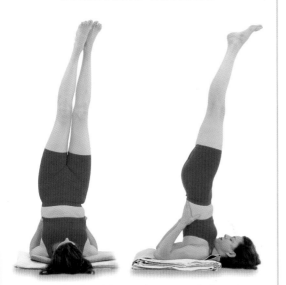

CORRECTING YOURSELF

If your legs tilt right or left in the final pose, bend your knees, move your waist aligning it with your chest, and straighten your legs again.

If your torso tilts forward, you will feel a heaviness in your chest and find it difficult to breathe. Push up your waist, thighs, hips, and buttocks.

6 Raise your feet toward the ceiling. Only the back of your neck, shoulders, and upper arms should rest on the blankets. Make sure that your body is perpendicular to the floor, from the shoulders to the knees.

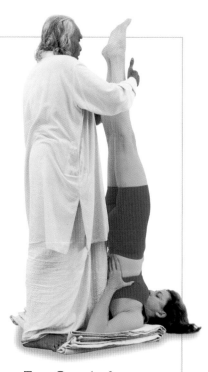

7 Press both palms into your back and straighten and stretch your body from the armpits to the toes. Your spine must be absolutely straight. Keep both elbows close to your body, as this keeps your chest expanded. To raise your torso further, release your palms, then press them into your back again. This will push your chest up further. Lift your body from the back of your neck, and not your throat. Push both shoulders back, to relax and stretch your neck. Extend your inner and outer legs toward the ceiling. Do not allow your legs to waver back and forth. Hold the pose for 2-3 minutes. Continue to breathe evenly.

THE GURU'S ADVICE

"Do not throw the legs back, but raise them slowly. Turn the inner calves outward and extend the skin of the outer legs up toward the heels."

Stretch your legs
from your groin
to your toes

Pull up your
pelvic rim

Keep your palms
close to your
shoulder blades

Keep your eyes
on your chest

Rest your elbows
squarely on the blankets

सालंब सर्वांगासन

Salamba Sarvangasana

ADVANCED WORK IN THE POSE

Create life in your spine. The energy in your spine should flow into your body through your fingers. Keep your eyes on your sternum, as this reinforces your will power and steadies your mind. Press your thumbs into the muscles of your back to push them toward the spine. This compresses the back. In the asana, your back should be narrow and your chest broad. Do not allow your elbows to spread outward. Bring them together, as too wide a distance between them makes your chest concave. Keep the bridge of your nose aligned with the middle of your sternum. Move your shoulders back. Focus on your inner legs, and stretch them toward the ceiling. This is a subtle and difficult action, but can be achieved over time. With practice, increase the duration of the pose to 5 minutes. Breathe evenly.

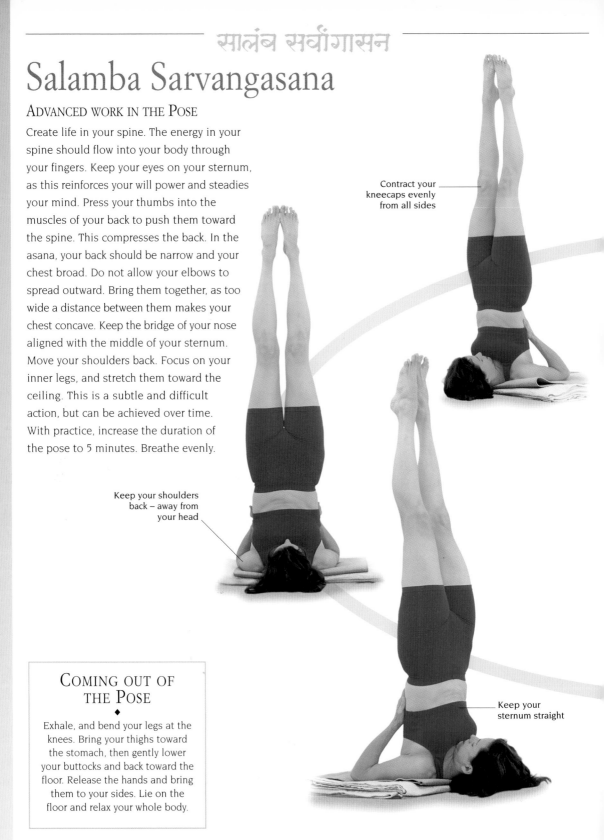

Contract your kneecaps evenly from all sides

Keep your shoulders back – away from your head

Keep your sternum straight

COMING OUT OF THE POSE

◆

Exhale, and bend your legs at the knees. Bring your thighs toward the stomach, then gently lower your buttocks and back toward the floor. Release the hands and bring them to your sides. Lie on the floor and relax your whole body.

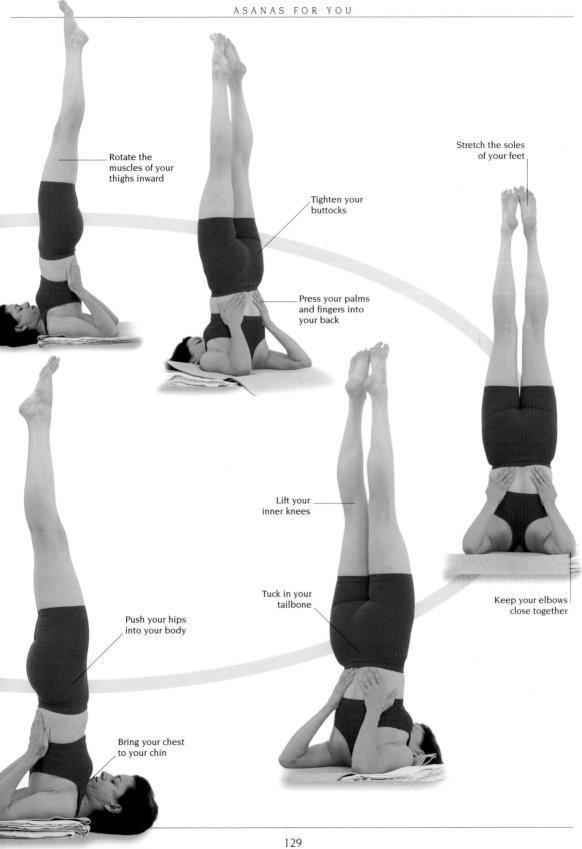

Rotate the muscles of your thighs inward

Tighten your buttocks

Press your palms and fingers into your back

Stretch the soles of your feet

Lift your inner knees

Tuck in your tailbone

Keep your elbows close together

Push your hips into your body

Bring your chest to your chin

SALAMBA SARVANGASANA – SHOULDERSTAND

हलासन

Halasana

- Plough pose -

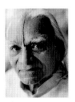

I N THIS ASANA, your body takes the shape of a plough – *hala* is the Sanskrit word for "plough". Practising Halasana regularly helps to increase your self-confidence and energy. The asana helps to restore calm and clarity of mind after a long illness. Halasana alleviates the effects of stress and strain by resting and relaxing your eyes and brain.

CAUTIONS
◆

Do not practise this asana if you have ischaemia, cervical spondylosis, or diarrhoea. Avoid this pose during menstruation. If you are prone to headaches, migraine, asthma, breathing difficulties, high blood pressure, physical and mental fatigue, or are overweight, practise Halasana with props and with your eyes closed.

1 Place two folded blankets, covered by a mat, on the floor. Lie down with your back, neck, and shoulders resting on the blankets. Keep your legs stretched out and tightened at the knees. Focus on your inner legs and stretch from your thighs to your heels. Place your arms by your sides, with your palms flat on the floor.

Rest your head on the floor

Extend the arches of your feet upward

3 Raise your hips and buttocks toward the ceiling in a smooth, rolling action. Bring your knees close to your chin and raise your lower legs, until your shins are perpendicular to the floor.

NOTE Once you have raised your buttocks off the floor, you may want to ask a helper to hold your ankles and push your legs toward your head.

Keep your knees together

2 Exhale, lift your buttocks off the floor, and bring your knees to your chest. Keep your arms straight and press your fingers firmly down on the floor. Push your shoulders back and broaden your chest.

Interlock your fingers firmly

Straighten and stretch your arms

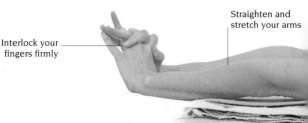

BENEFITS

Relieves fatigue and boosts energy levels

Controls hypertension

Rejuvenates the abdominal organs and improves digestion

Lengthens the spine, and improves its alignment

Helps to treat hernia and haemorrhoids, if practised with legs separated

Relieves pain or cramps in fingers, hands, wrists, elbows, and shoulders, if practised with arms and interlocked fingers extended toward the legs

4 Bend your elbows. Place your hands on the small of your back (*see inset*). Raise your hips and buttocks even further, until your torso is perpendicular to the floor and your thighs are positioned above your face. Bring your bent knees over your forehead, before you lower your legs to the floor. Breathe evenly.

Keep your feet, knees, and thighs together

Relax your facial skin and muscles

5 Swing your hips and buttocks over your head, until they are perpendicular to the floor and in line with your shoulders. Slowly straighten your legs, and lower them until your toes rest on the floor. Raise your chest, bringing your sternum to touch your chin. Stretch your arms out behind your back on the blankets. Then interlock your fingers firmly at the knuckles, rotating your wrists until your hands point toward the ceiling. Stay in the pose for 1-5 minutes. Breathe evenly.

NOTE Initially, you may stretch your arms out toward your feet. Once you are comfortable in this pose, stretch your arms out behind your back.

Tighten your buttocks

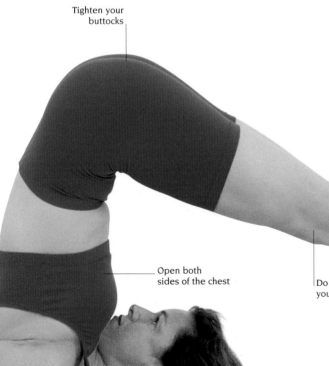

Open both sides of the chest

Do not bend your knees

Press your toes down on the floor

हलासन

Halasana

ADVANCED WORK IN THE POSE

As you hold this pose, make sure that your brain is not tense. Consciously relax the skin and muscles of your face. Keep your gaze on your chest – do not look up. Drop your eyes down in their sockets, as this helps to relax the facial muscles. Your neck should be completely soft, as this rests the brain. Remember that your throat is the site of the Vishuddhi *chakra* (*see page* 37). If it tightens, your brain will become tense. Lift your sternum and chest to relax your throat and ensure smooth and effortless breathing. Increase the space between your navel and diaphragm.

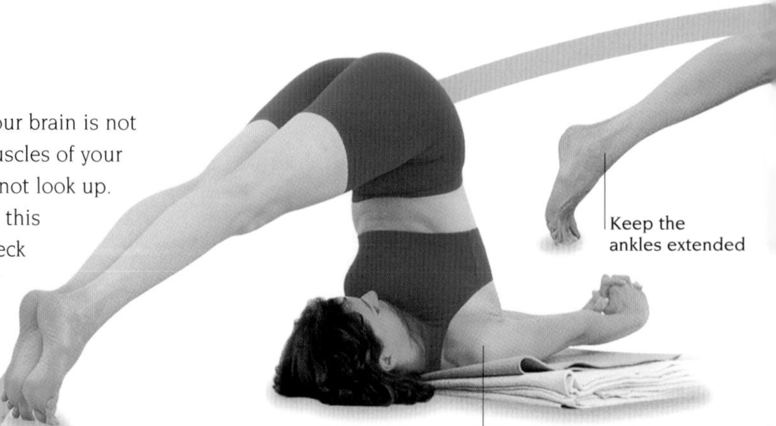

Keep the ankles extended

Push your shoulders into your body

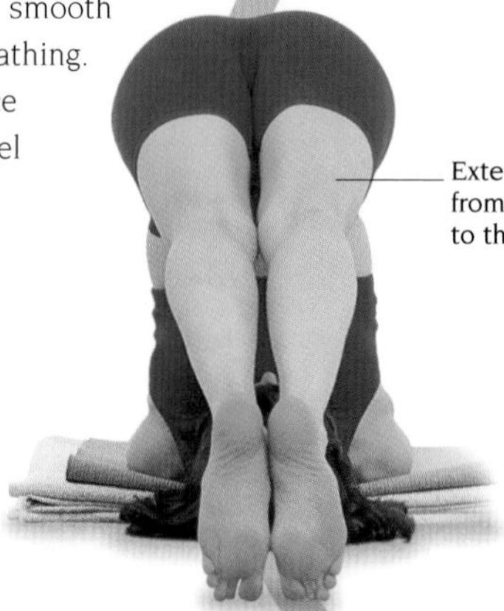

Extend your legs from the buttocks to the heels

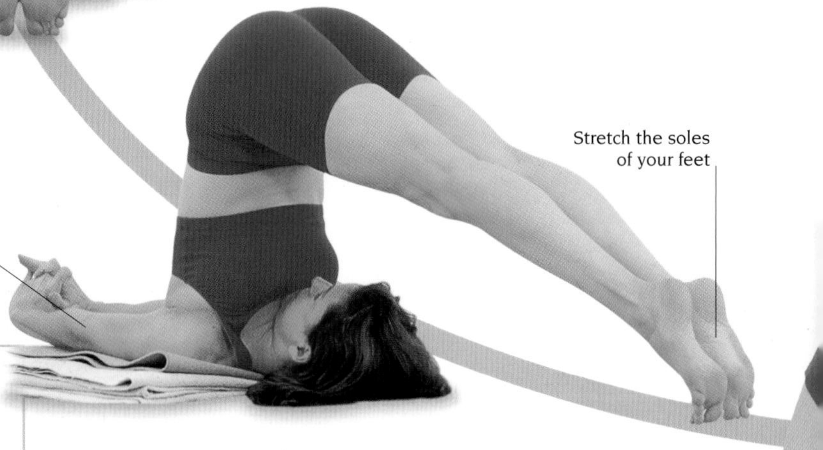

Stretch the soles of your feet

Press the arms downward

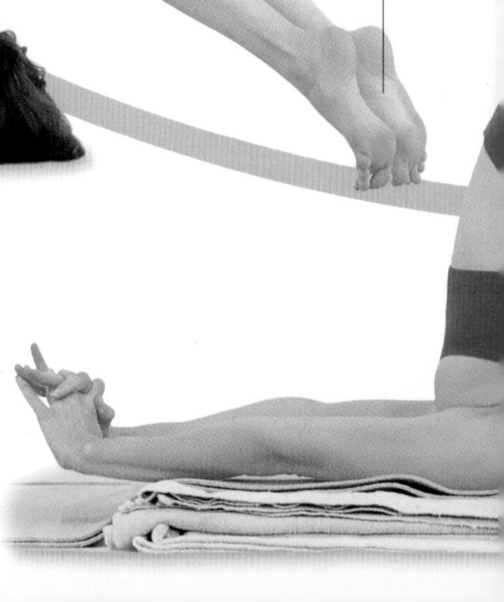

COMING OUT OF THE POSE

◆

Slowly, and with control, lift your legs off the floor. Bring your thighs and knees toward your stomach. Push your buttocks back and lower them to the floor. Flatten your back and relax your entire body, breathing deeply.

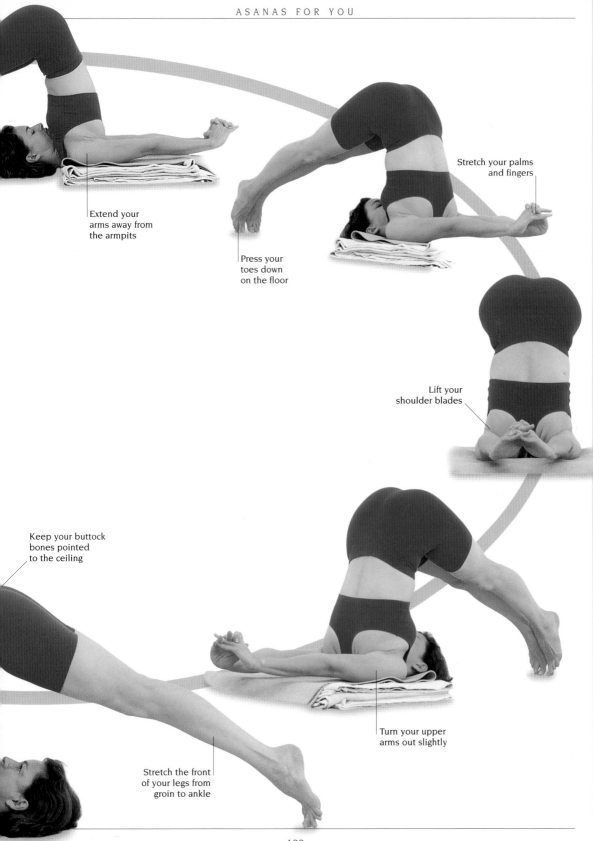

Extend your
arms away from
the armpits

Press your
toes down
on the floor

Stretch your palms
and fingers

Lift your
shoulder blades

Keep your buttock
bones pointed
to the ceiling

Turn your upper
arms out slightly

Stretch the front
of your legs from
groin to ankle

Back Bends

"Asanas penetrate deep into each layer of the body and ultimately into the consciousness itself."

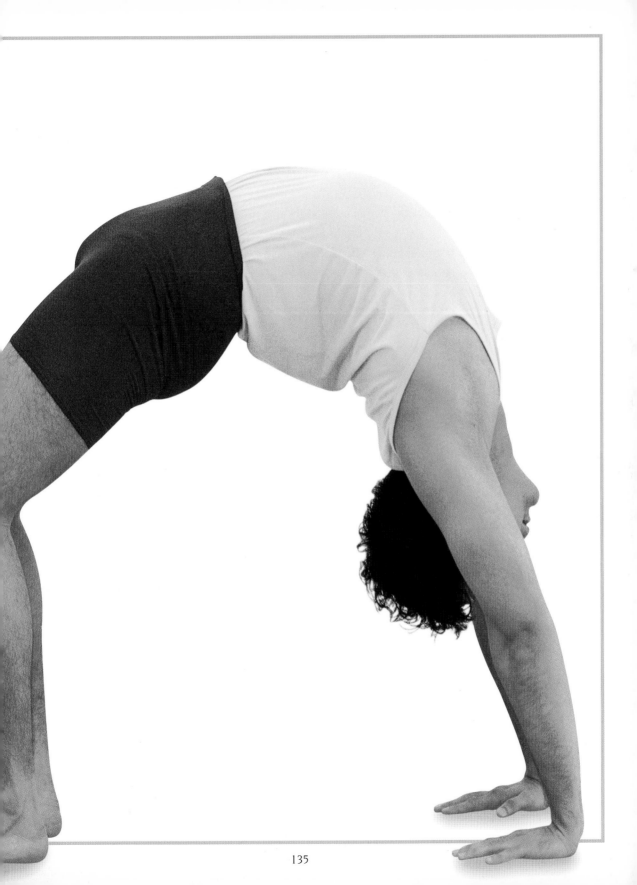

उष्ट्रासन

Ustrasana

- Camel pose -

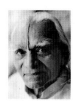

IN THIS ASANA, you bend back until the shape of your body resembles that of a camel – *ustra* means "camel" in Sanskrit. Ustrasana is recommended for beginners, as well as for the elderly, because the balance of the final pose is relatively easy to attain. The asana also helps people in sedentary occupations, whose work entails bending forward for long periods. Practising the asana regularly will relieve stiffness in the back, shoulders, and ankles.

CAUTIONS

◆

Do not practise this asana if you have severe constipation, diarrhoea, headaches, migraine, or hypertension. If you are recovering from a heart attack, practise Ustrasana with props (*see page* 45).

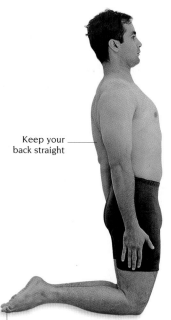

Keep your back straight

Rest your toes on the floor

1 Kneel on the floor with your arms by your sides. Keep your thighs, knees, and feet together. Rest on the front of your feet, with the toes pointing to the back. Keep your torso upright and breathe evenly.

NOTE If keeping your knees together leads to a feeling of strain in your thighs, practise with your knees slightly apart. This also allows for a freer movement of the spine.

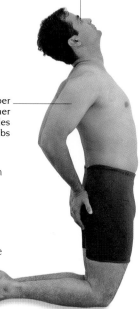

Keep your eyes open

Move your upper arms closer together and the shoulder blades in toward the back ribs

2 Exhale, and place your palms on your buttocks. Push your thighs forward slightly and then pull them up toward your groin. Push your spine into your body. Then, gradually bend your back, and lower it toward the floor. Simultaneously, extend your ribcage and broaden your chest. Continue to breathe evenly.

BENEFITS

◆

Helps to correct posture

◆

Increases lung capacity

◆

Improves blood circulation to all the organs of the body

◆

Tones the muscles of the back and spine

◆

Removes stiffness in the shoulders, back, and ankles

◆

Relieves abdominal cramps

◆

Regulates menstrual flow

3 Push your shoulders back and stretch your arms from your shoulders toward your feet. Inhale, throw your head back, and hold both heels with your hands. Make sure that your thighs are perpendicular to the floor. Push your spine down toward your legs and breathe evenly.

NOTE Initially, you may hold one heel at a time by tilting each shoulder individually.

Expand your chest

4 Push your feet down on the floor. At the same time, press down on your soles with your palms. Your fingers should point toward your toes (*see inset*). Tighten your buttocks and pull in your tailbone. Push your shoulder blades back. Take your head as far back as possible, but take care not to strain your throat. Stay in the pose for 30 seconds.

Lift your sternum

Do not tilt your head too far back

Pull your spine into your body

Slide your hands over the heels to cover your soles fully

Keep your quadricep muscles stretched

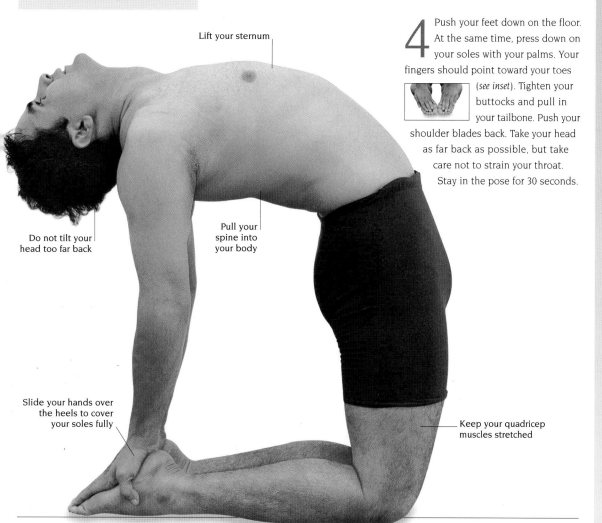

उष्ट्रासन

Ustrasana

ADVANCED WORK IN THE POSE

Push your shins down on the floor, and press your palms down on your soles. Lift and stretch the length of your spine, so that your body forms an arch. Your chest, armpits, and back should coil inward, as this will support the back of your chest. Consciously suck in your back ribs, and feel your kidneys being drawn in and squeezed. Try to create a space first between the dome of the diaphragm and the navel; and second, between the navel and the groin. By doing this, you will be extending your abdominal and pelvic organs, as well as your intestines. Roll the inner sides of your upper arms to the front and the outer sides of your upper arms to the back. Keep your elbow joints locked. Breathe evenly.

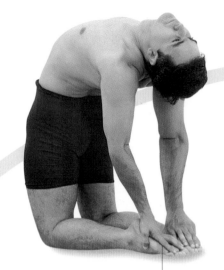

Keep the front of your feet on the floor

Lock your elbows

Do not strain your throat

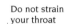

Press your palms on your feet and extend the arms toward their sockets

COMING OUT OF THE POSE

◆

Exhale, and lessen the pressure of your palms on the feet. Raise your torso, keeping your arms by your sides. The impetus for the upward movement should come from the thighs and chest. If you cannot raise both your arms together, lift them, one by one.

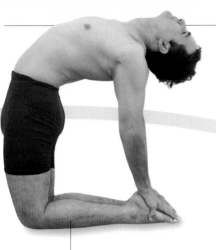

Keep your chest
raised and expanded

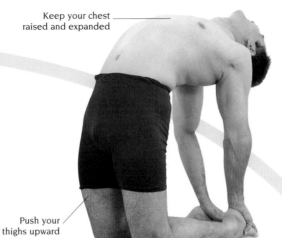

Extend and press
your shins to
the floor

Push your
thighs upward

Stretch the
abdominal muscles

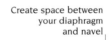

Create space between
your diaphragm
and navel

Push your
collar bones back

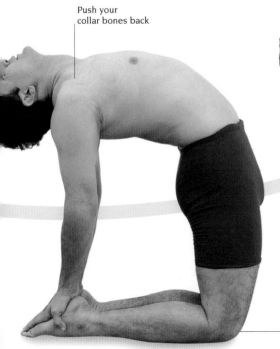

139

ऊर्ध्व धनुरासन
Urdhva Dhanurasana

- Bow pose -

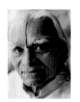

YOUR BODY ARCHES back to form an extended bow in this asana. U*rdhva* means "upward" in Sanskrit, while *dhanur* translates as "bow". Regular practice of Urdhva Dhanurasana keeps your body supple, and creates a feeling of vitality and lightness. The asana stimulates the adrenal glands, strengthening your will power, and increasing your capacity to bear stress.

CAUTIONS

◆

Do not practise this asana if your blood pressure is too high or too low. Avoid this pose if you have constipation or if you have diarrhoea. Avoid this pose when you are feeling tired. Do not practise during an attack of migraine or a severe headache. Avoid this pose if you have a cardiac condition or ischaemia.

Press your thighs and calves together

Press your palms on the floor and keep your elbows pointed forward

1 Lie on your back on the floor. Bend both knees and pull your heels to your buttocks. Spread your feet, so that they align with your hips. Bend your elbows and bring them over your head. Place your palms on the floor, on either side of your head. Your fingers should point toward your shoulders.

NOTE At first, you may find it difficult to bring your heels close to your buttocks. Use your hands to pull the feet into position.

2 Focus on your palms and feet, as you are going to use them to launch your pose. Pull your shoulder blades up, and the muscles of your back into your body. Exhale, then lift your torso and buttocks off the floor. Breathe evenly.

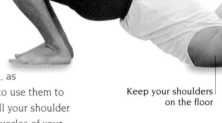

Ensure that your elbows are shoulder-width apart

Keep your shoulders on the floor

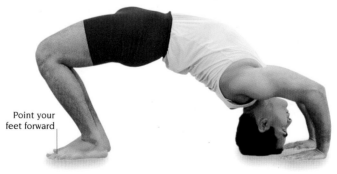

Point your feet forward

3 Lift your chest and place the crown of your head on the floor. Take two breaths. Exhale sharply, and suck in your back and buttocks. Shift your weight from your palms to the front of your feet, and push up your torso in one single movement. Adjust your pose until your weight is equally distributed on your arms and legs.

BENEFITS

◆

Prevents the arteries of the heart from thickening, and ensures healthy blood circulation throughout the body

◆

Tones the spine

◆

Strengthens the abdominal and pelvic organs

◆

Stimulates the pituitary, pineal, and thyroid glands

◆

Prevents prolapse of the uterus

◆

Helps to prevent excess menstrual flow and eases menstrual cramps

THE GURU'S ADVICE

"Do not merely push your chest forward, as this alone will not prevent the arch of the torso from collapsing. Look at how I am lifting the sides of my student's lower ribcage. You must lift both sides of your chest up toward the ceiling."

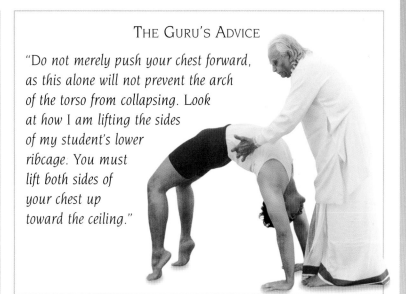

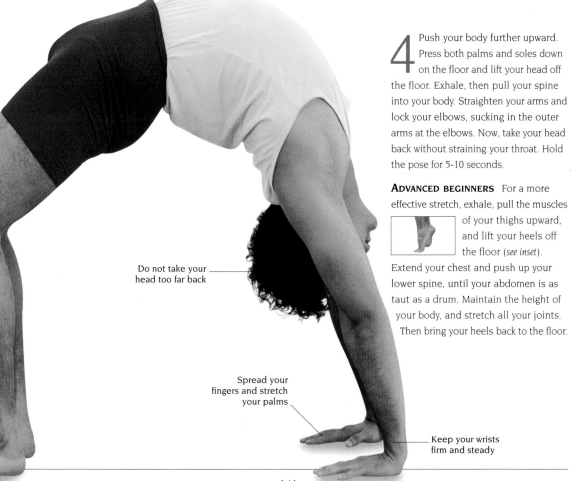

Do not take your head too far back

Spread your fingers and stretch your palms

Keep your wrists firm and steady

4 Push your body further upward. Press both palms and soles down on the floor and lift your head off the floor. Exhale, then pull your spine into your body. Straighten your arms and lock your elbows, sucking in the outer arms at the elbows. Now, take your head back without straining your throat. Hold the pose for 5-10 seconds.

ADVANCED BEGINNERS For a more effective stretch, exhale, pull the muscles of your thighs upward, and lift your heels off the floor (*see inset*). Extend your chest and push up your lower spine, until your abdomen is as taut as a drum. Maintain the height of your body, and stretch all your joints. Then bring your heels back to the floor.

ऊर्ध्व धनुरासन

Urdhva Dhanurasana

ADVANCED WORK IN THE POSE

In the final pose, your body stretches in two directions: one from the palms, and the other from the feet. The meeting point is at the base of the spine. Try to raise this point higher and higher. Open up the spaces between the ribs, especially at the bottom of your chest. Broaden your diaphragm. Suck in your shoulder blades and back ribs – imagine you are squeezing your kidneys. Make sure your weight is evenly distributed on your hands and feet, and your arms and legs are extended (pulled up) toward the ceiling. Initially, hold the pose for 5-10 seconds, breathing evenly With practice, repeat the asana 3 to 5 times. This will bring greater freedom of movement to your body and improve the effectiveness of your stretch.

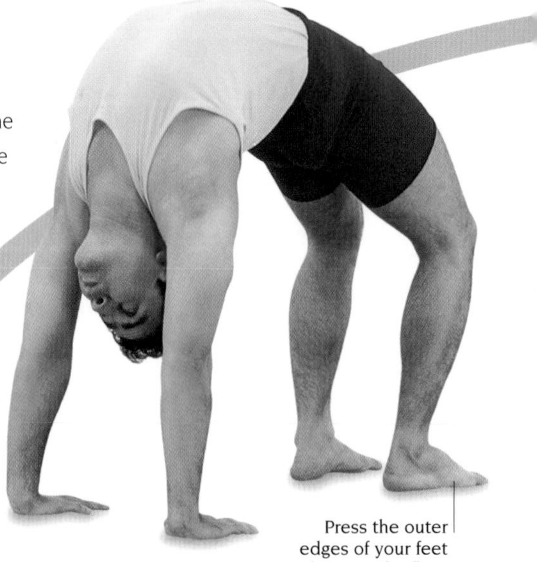

Press the outer edges of your feet down on the floor

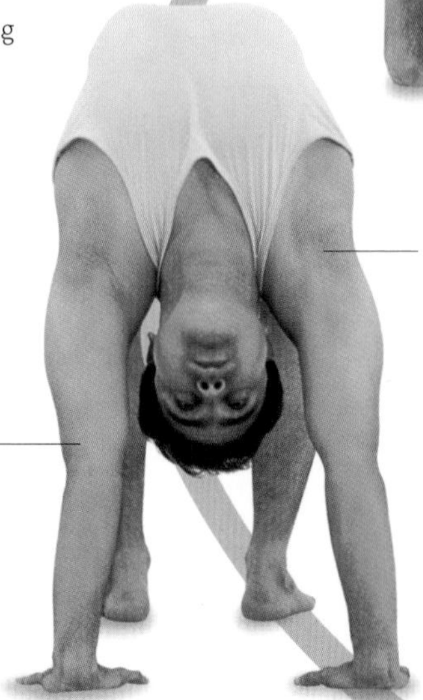

Open out your armpits

Stretch your arms from the wrists to the armpits

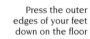

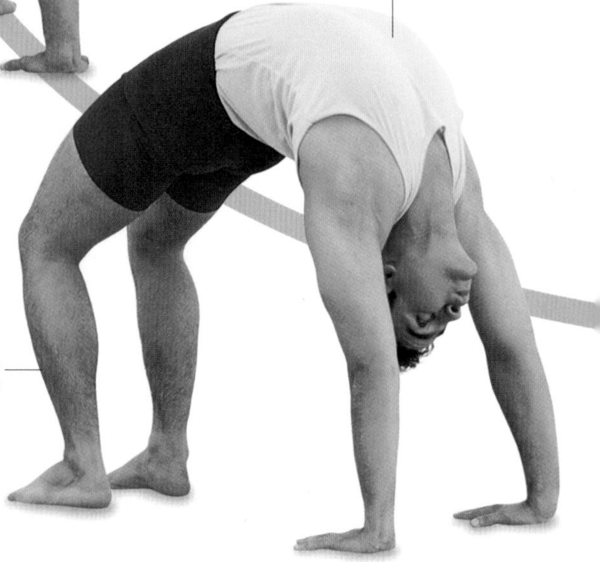

Move your chest toward the ceiling

Pull your shins up toward your thighs

COMING OUT OF THE POSE
◆

Exhale, and bend your elbows and knees. Lower your torso, then bring the crown of your head down to the floor. Lower your back and buttocks to the floor. Lie on your back and take a few breaths.

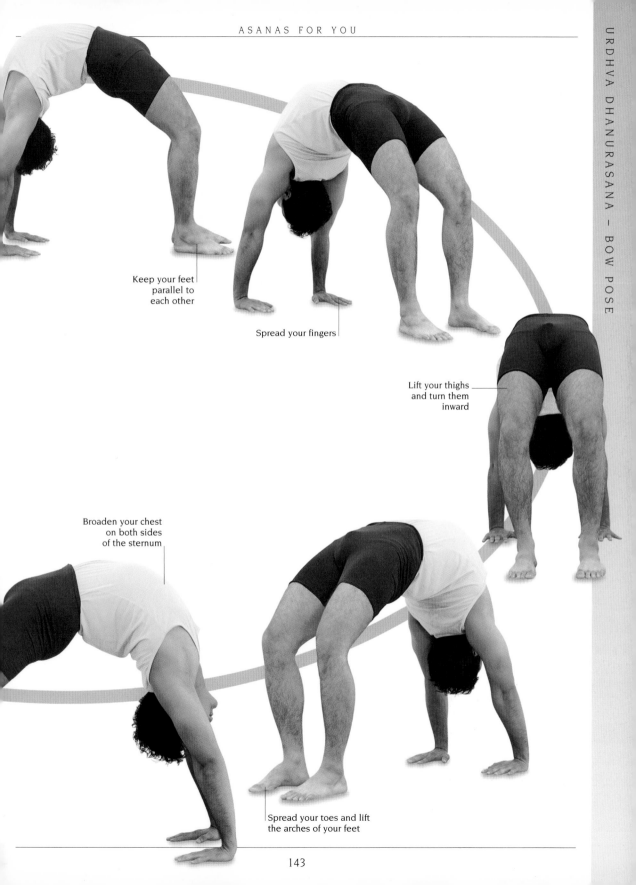

Keep your feet parallel to each other

Spread your fingers

Lift your thighs and turn them inward

Broaden your chest on both sides of the sternum

Spread your toes and lift the arches of your feet

Reclining Asanas

"Feel the inner mind touching your entire body – even the remotest parts where the mind does not normally reach."

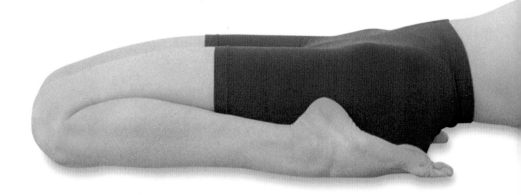

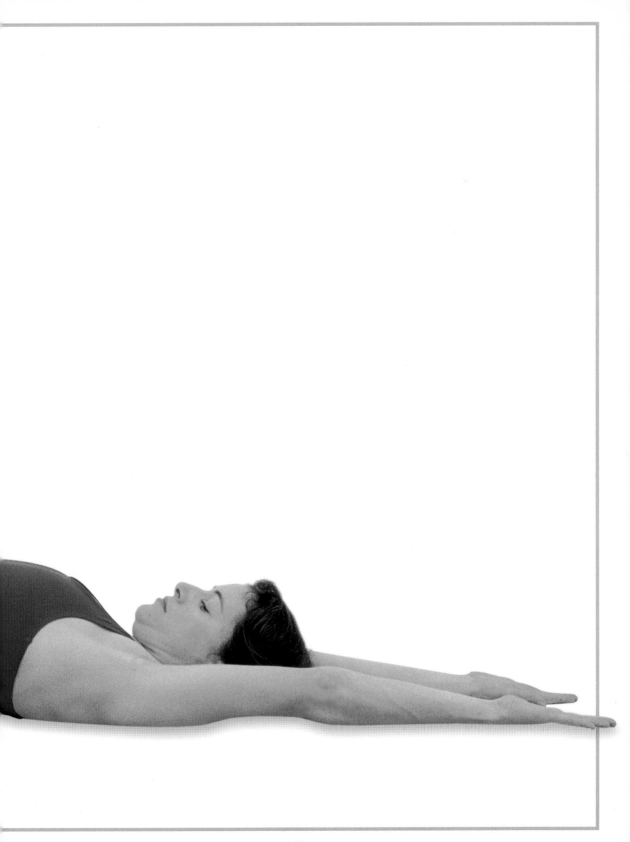

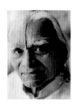

सुप्त वीरासन

Supta Virasana

- Reclining hero stretch -

THIS IS A VARIATION OF the sitting pose, Virasana (*see page* 84). In this asana, you rest your torso on the floor. *Supta* means "lying down" in Sanskrit, while *vira* translates as "hero" or "champion". Athletes, and all those who are on their feet for long periods, will find this asana helpful, as the legs receive an intense and invigorating stretch. If you practise this pose last thing at night, your legs will feel rested and rejuvenated in the morning.

CAUTIONS

◆

Do not practise this asana if you have a cardiac condition, lower backache, or osteoarthritis of the knees. Those with gout, arthritis of the ankles, or spinal disc disorders should practise with props (*see page* 45). Women should place a bolster under the back during menstruation

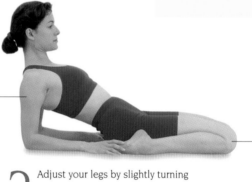

Press your forearms and extend the chest

Ensure that your knees remain together

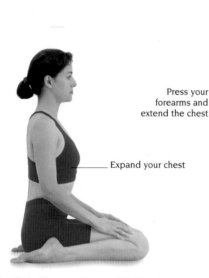

Expand your chest

2 Adjust your legs by slightly turning in your thighs and turning out your calves. Exhale, and lower your back gradually toward the floor. Rest your elbows, one by one, on the floor. Keep your palms on the bottom of your feet. Breathe evenly.

1 Sit in Virasana (*see page* 84). Keep both knees together and spread your feet about 0.5m (18in) apart, until they rest beside your hips. To avoid strain, ensure that the inner side of each calf touches the outer side of each thigh. Turn your soles toward the ceiling. Each of your toes should rest on the floor. Stretch your ankles fully and extend the soles toward the toes. Let the energy flow in both directions through your feet.

Turn the thighs in and press them down

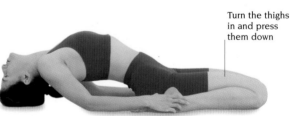

3 Place the crown of your head on the floor. Now, lower your shoulders and upper torso to rest your head, and then your back, on the floor. Stretch your arms along your sides. Press your wrists against your soles.

BENEFITS

◆

Helps to reduce cardiac disorders

◆

Stretches the abdomen, back, and waist

◆

Relieves rheumatism and pain in the upper and middle back

◆

Aids digestion after a heavy meal

◆

Soothes acidity and stomach ulcers

◆

Relieves the symptoms of asthma

◆

Reduces menstrual pain, and helps treat disorders of the ovaries

THE GURU'S ADVICE

"Do not push your buttocks toward the spine, since this causes your lumbar spine to arch. Look at how I am pushing my student's waist and buttocks toward her knees. You must lengthen your buttock muscles and allow the lumbar spine to extend. Then rest the spine on the floor."

4 Move your elbows out to the sides and lie flat on the floor, until the spine is fully extended. Bring your head down and spread your shoulders away from your neck. Rest your shoulder blades and knees on the floor.

Turn the heels out by holding them with your palms

5 Take your arms over your head and stretch them out behind you on the floor, with your palms facing the ceiling. Ensure that both shoulder blades remain flat on the floor and do not let your buttocks or knees lift off the floor. Release your back and allow it to descend completely to the floor. If your back arches, it causes stress to the lower back. Press your thighs together, taking care not to jerk your knees. Breathe evenly and stay in the pose for 30-60 seconds.

Expand your chest evenly on either side of the sternum

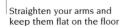

Straighten your arms and keep them flat on the floor

Rotate the outer edges of your feet toward the floor

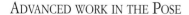

Supta Virasana

ADVANCED WORK IN THE POSE

In the final pose, the stretch of your arms pulls your thighs and abdomen toward your chest – massaging them in the process. Move both shoulder blades in, and open your chest fully. Press your shoulders down, ensuring that your knees and buttocks remain on the floor. The front and the back of your body should be evenly elongated and your armpits fully stretched. Push your pelvis toward the knees and press it down on the floor. Focus on your ribs. Consciously extend them toward your head. Gradually, increase the time spent in the pose to 5-7 minutes.

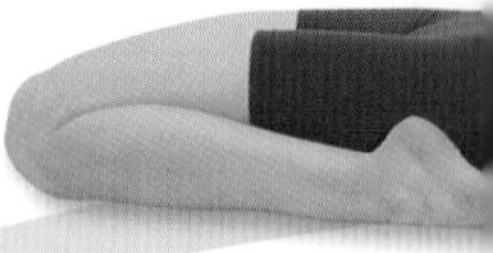

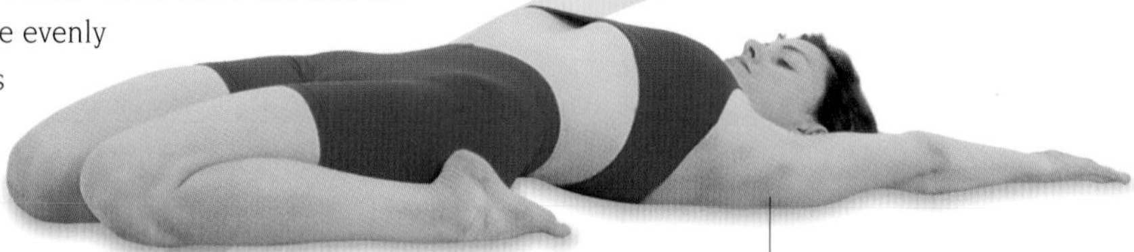

Tuck in your shoulder blades

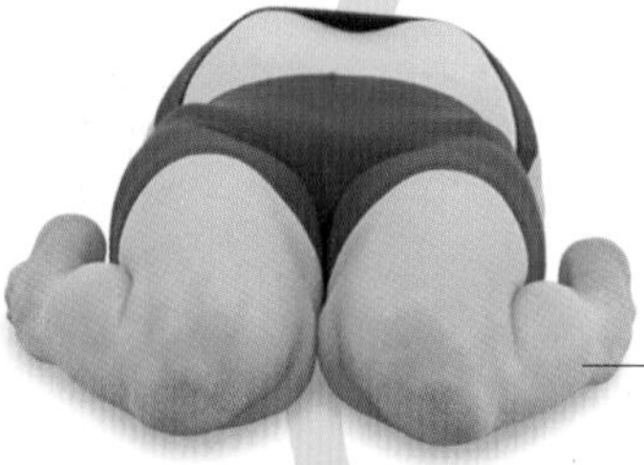

Press your shins down on the floor

Push your thighs together

"When th

and still, wh

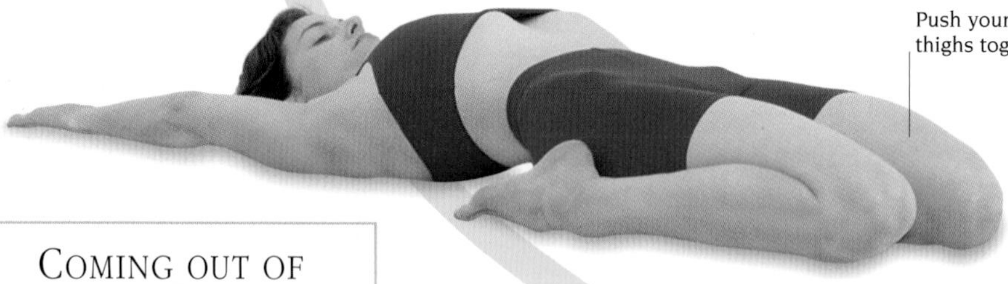

COMING OUT OF THE POSE
◆

Bring your hands over your head and hold your ankles. Lift your head and torso off the floor, supporting yourself on your elbows. Sit up in Virasana. Exhale and straighten your legs, one at a time. Sit in Dandasana.

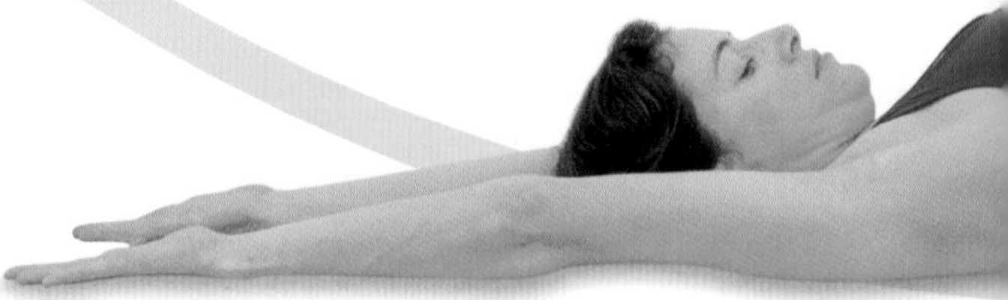

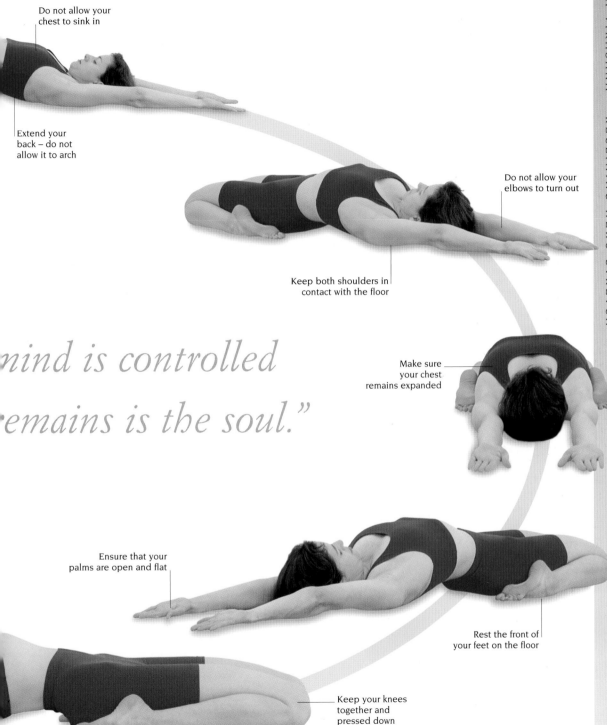

Do not allow your chest to sink in

Extend your back – do not allow it to arch

Do not allow your elbows to turn out

Keep both shoulders in contact with the floor

Make sure your chest remains expanded

nind is controlled

emains is the soul."

Ensure that your palms are open and flat

Rest the front of your feet on the floor

Keep your knees together and pressed down

शवासन

Savasana

- Corpse pose -

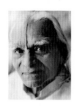

I N THIS ASANA, the body is kept as motionless as a corpse and the mind is alert, yet calm. The word *sava* means "corpse" in Sanskrit. Savasana removes fatigue and soothes the mind. Each part of the body is positioned properly to achieve total relaxation. When you practise this asana, your organs of perception – the eyes, ears, and tongue – withdraw from the outside world. The body and the mind become one, and you experience inner silence. This asana is the first step in the practice of meditation.

CAUTIONS
♦

If you are pregnant, have a respiratory ailment, or experience anxiety, practise Savasana with your head and chest raised on a bolster If you have a backache, lie with your back on the floor, and rest your calves on the seat of a chair, with your thighs perpendicular to the floor. Do not practise Savasana between other asanas.

Press the backs of your knees to the floor

Spread the collar bones out to the sides

Keep the head straight – do not tilt it to one side

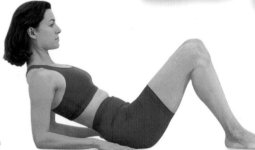

1 Sit in Dandasana (*see page 82*). Push the flesh of your buttocks out to the sides, so that your weight is equally distributed on both buttock bones. Breathe evenly.

Ensure that your back is straight

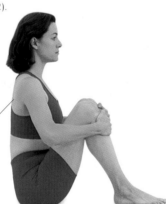

2 Bend your knees and bring your heels closer to the buttocks. Hold the tops of your shins and press your buttock bones down on the floor. Check that your back is straight.

3 To lower your torso toward the floor, place your forearms and palms on the floor and lean back on your elbows. Do not move your feet, knees, or buttocks.

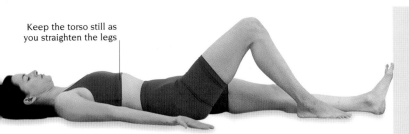

Keep the torso still as you straighten the legs

BENEFITS

◆

Helps to alleviate nervous tension, migraine, insomnia, and chronic fatigue syndrome

◆

Relaxes the body and eases breathing

◆

Soothes the nervous system and brings peace of mind

◆

Enhances recovery from all long-term or serious illnesses

4 Lower your torso to the floor, vertebra by vertebra, until the back of your head rests on the floor. Turn your palms to face the ceiling. Close your eyes, then straighten your legs, one by one.

ADVANCED BEGINNERS Stretch your torso away from your hips to straighten the spine. Extend the spine fully and keep it flat on the floor. Make sure that the stretch along the legs and the torso is equal on both sides of the body.

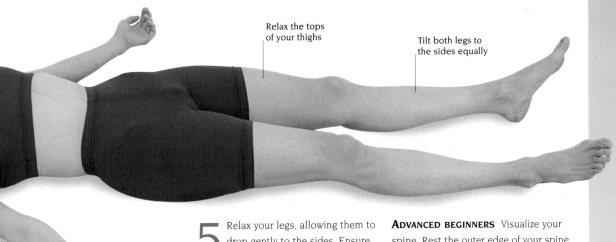

Relax the tops of your thighs

Tilt both legs to the sides equally

Relax the fingers and the centres of the palms

5 Relax your legs, allowing them to drop gently to the sides. Ensure that your kneecaps drop to the sides equally. Move your arms away from your torso without raising your shoulders off the floor. Push your collar bones out to the sides. Keep your eyes closed and focus on your breathing. Stay in this pose for 5-7 minutes.

ADVANCED BEGINNERS Visualize your spine. Rest the outer edge of your spine comfortably on the floor. Expand your chest out to the sides and relax your sternum. Focus on your diaphragm – it should be absolutely free of tension. As you push your collar bones out to the sides, allow your neck to dip to the floor. Relax the muscles of your neck.

Savasana

ADVANCED WORK IN THE POSE

As your neck dips to the floor (*see Step 5, page* 151), you will feel a soothing sensation in the back of your brain. When this area of the brain relaxes, move on to the front of the brain. From the crown of the head, the energy should descend in a spiral action toward the bridge of the nose, and down to a point located at the sternum. When the energy reaches this point, the three layers and five sheaths that comprise your body (*see page* 24) come together and are integrated into a single, harmonious whole. This is the ultimate aim of Savasana.

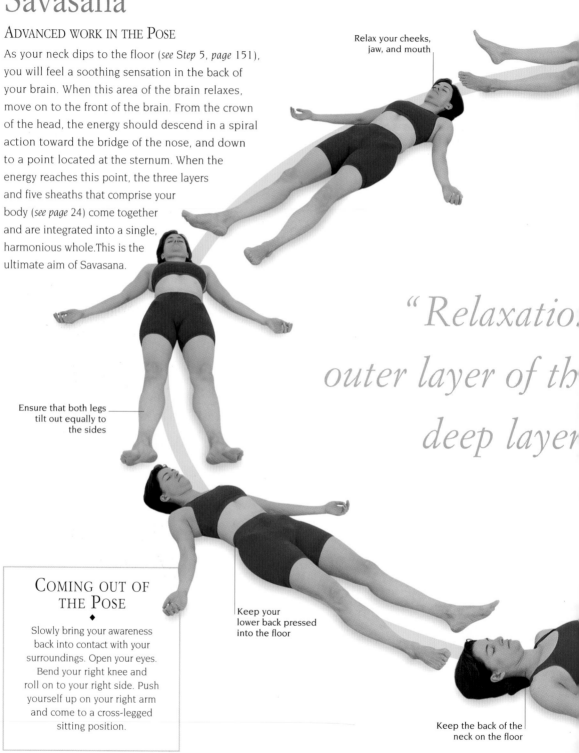

Relax your cheeks, jaw, and mouth

Ensure that both legs tilt out equally to the sides

"*Relaxatio.*

outer layer of th

deep layer

COMING OUT OF THE POSE

◆

Slowly bring your awareness back into contact with your surroundings. Open your eyes. Bend your right knee and roll on to your right side. Push yourself up on your right arm and come to a cross-legged sitting position.

Keep your lower back pressed into the floor

Keep the back of the neck on the floor

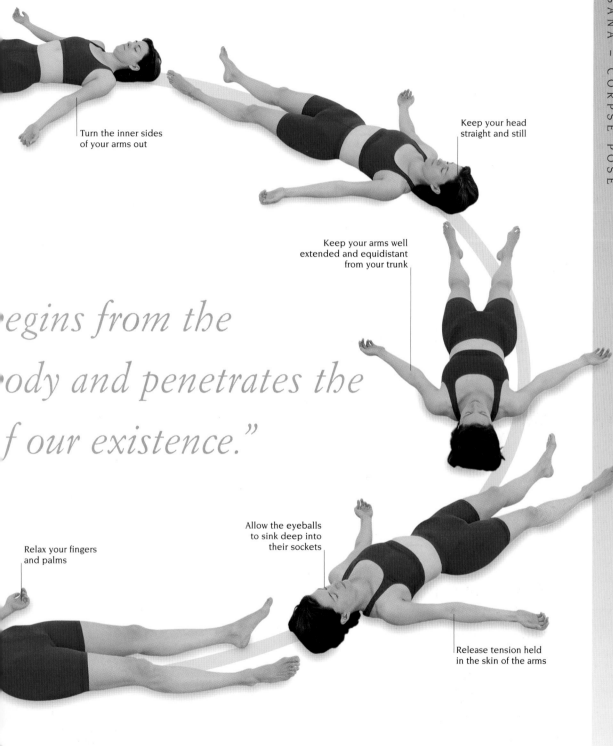

Turn the inner sides
of your arms out

Keep your head
straight and still

Keep your arms well
extended and equidistant
from your trunk

egins from the

ody and penetrates the

f our existence."

Allow the eyeballs
to sink deep into
their sockets

Relax your fingers
and palms

Release tension held
in the skin of the arms

Glossary

Abhyantara inhalation

Ahankara false pride

Ahimsa creed of non-violence

Ajna chakra energy or command chakra

Alabdha bhumikatva indisposition

Alasya laziness

Anahata chakra spiritual heart chakra

Anandamaya kosha the sheath of bliss, the most important of the 5 sheaths of the body, reached by the practice of yoga

Angamejayatva unsteadiness in the body

Annamaya kosha anatomical sheath, one of 5 sheaths of the body

Antara-kumbhaka suspension of breath with full lungs

Antaranga-sadhana emotional and mental discipline gained through following the 8 limbs or steps of yoga

Antaratma-sadhana quest for the soul gained through following the 8 limbs or steps of yoga

Anusasanam discipline

Aparigraha freedom from desire

Arambhavastha beginners' stage of yoga, practised at the level of the physical body alone

Asmita egoism

Astanga yoga eight limbs: the steps to self-realization through the practice of yoga

Asteya freedom from avarice

Atman the self or soul

Avirati desire for sensual satisfaction

Ayama expansion or distribution of energy

Bahya exhalation

Bahya-kumbhaka suspension of breath with empty lungs

Bahiranga-sadhana one of 3 yogic disciplines, comprising the practice of ethics

Bhakti marg path of love and devotion

Bharadvaja a sage, the father of the warrior Dronacharya

Bharanti darshana false knowledge

Brahmacharya chastity

Buddhi intelligence

Chitta the restraint of consciousness

Chittavritti an imbalance in the mental state

Chakras critical junctions in the body, notionally located along the spine,

which, when activated by asanas and pranayama, transform cosmic energy into spiritual energy

Dharana concentration, the sixth limb or step of Astanga yoga

Dhyana the seventh stage of the 8 limbs or steps of Astanga yoga

Dronacharya son of the sage Bharadvaja and a major character in the epic, *Mahabharata*

Dorsal region the upper part of the body, relating especially to the back

Duhkha misery or pain

Ekagra a focused state of mind

Floating ribs the last 2 pairs of ribs which are not attached to the sternum

Ghatavastha Intermediate stage of yoga, when the mind and body learn to move together

Gheranda Samhita text on yoga, written by the sage Gheranda in the 15th century

Guru teacher; one who hands down a system of knowledge to a disciple

Guru-sishya parampara the tradition of teaching, dating back centuries, of teacher and student

Hatha yoga sighting the soul through the restraint of energy

Hathayoga Pradipika treatise on yoga compiled in the 15th century by the sage Svatmarama

Isvara pranidhana devotion to God

Jivatma the individual self

Jnana marg path of knowledge whereby the seeker learns to discriminate between the real and the unreal

Kaivalya freedom of emancipation

Karma marg path of selfless service without thought of reward

Karana sharira causal body, one of the 3 layers of the body

Karya sharira gross body, one of the 3 layers of the body

Kathopanishad ancient text circa 300-400 BC

Klesha sorrow caused by egoism, desire, attachment, and hatred

Ksipta a distracted mind

Kundalini divine, cosmic energy which is latent in every human being

Kumbhaka retention of energy

Manas the mind

Manava (manusya) an intelligent and conscious human being

Mahabharata the most ancient of the Indian epics, dating to the first millennium BC

Manipuraka chakra site of the sense of fear and apprehension

Manomaya kosha psychological sheath, one of the 5 sheaths of the body

Marichi a sage, son of Brahma, the creator of the universe

Menorrhagia abnormally heavy or long periods

Mudha a dull, inert mind

Muladhara chakra controls sexual energy

Nadi notional channels which distribute energy from the chakras through the body

Nirbija seedless

Niruddha a controlled and restrained mind

Nishpattyavastha ultimate stage of yoga practice, the state of perfection

Niyama self-restraint

Parmatama the universal self

Parichayavastha third stage of yoga practice, when the intelligence and the body become one

Parigraha possessiveness

Patanjali, a sage, the founder of yoga; believed to have lived sometime between 300 BC-AD 300

Patanjala Yoga Darshana corpus of aphorisms on yoga, compiled between 300 BC-AD 300 and usually attributed to the sage Patanjali

Perineum the area between the thighs, behind the genital organs and in front of the anus

Pramada indifference

Prakriti shakti energy of nature

Prana vital energy or life-force

Pranamaya kosha life-force sheath, one of the 5 sheaths of the body

Pranayama control of energy through breathing

Pratyahara mental detachment from the external world

Psoriasis an ailment leading to dry and scaly patches on the skin

Purusha shakti energy of the soul

Raja yoga sighting the soul through the restraint of consciousness

Rajasic spicy, pungent foods that overstimulate the body and mind

Sahasrara chakra the most important chakra which, when uncoiled, brings the seeker to freedom

Samadhi self-realization

Samshaya doubt

Samyama integration of the body, breath, mind, intellect, and self

Santosha contentment

Sarvaanga sadhana holistic practice which integrates the body, mind and the self

Sattvic natural, organic vegetarian food

Satya truth

Saucha cleanliness

Scoliosis a curved spine

Shakti vital energy and the sense of self,

which determine a person's emotions, will power and discrimination

Shvasa-prashvasa uneven respiration or unsteadiness

Styana reluctance to work

Suksma sharira the subtle body, one of the 3 layers of the body

Svadhyaya to study one's body, mind, intellect, and ego

Svatmarama sage, author of *Hathayoga Pradipika*

Swadhishtana chakra site of worldly desires

Tamasic food containing meat or alcohol

Tapas austerity gained through the committed practice of yoga

Vijnanamaya kosha intellectual sheath, one of the 5 sheaths of the body

Viksipta a scattered, fearful mind

Virabhadra a legendary warrior

Vishuddhi chakra seat of intellectual awareness

Vyadhi physical ailments

Yama ethical codes for daily life

Yoga the path which integrates the body, senses, mind, and the intelligence, with the self

Yogacharya a teacher and a master of yogic traditions

Yoga-agni the fire of yoga which, when lit, ignites the kundalini

Yogabhrastha falling from the grace of yoga

Yoga marg the journey to self-realization, when the mind and its actions are brought under control

Yoga Sutras a collection of aphorisms on the practice of yoga, attributed to the sage Patanjali

Yogi a student, a seeker of truth

Names of Asanas

Name	Translation
Adhomukha Svanasana	Downward-facing dog stretch
Baddhakonasana	Fixed angle pose
Bharadvajasana	Lateral twist of the spine; name of the sage
Dandasana	Staff pose
Halasana	Plough pose
Janu Sirsasana	Head on knee pose
Marichyasana	lateral twist of the spine; name of the sage
Parsvottanasana	Intense torso stretch
Paschimottanasana	Intense back stretch
Salamba Sarvangasana	Shoulderstand
Salamba Sirsasana	Headstand
Savasana	Corpse pose
Supta Virasana	Reclining hero pose
Tadasana	Mountain pose
Trianga Mukhaikapada Paschimottanasana	Three parts of the body stretch
Urdhva Dhanurasana	Bow pose
Ustrasana	Camel pose
Uttanasana	Intense forward stretch
Utthita Parsvakonasana	Intense side stretch
Utthita Trikonasana	Extended triangle pose
Virabhadrasana 1	Warrior pose 1
Virabhadrasana 2	Warrior pose 2
Virasana	Hero pose

Index

Acknowledgments

PUBLISHER'S ACKNOWLEDGMENTS

Dorling Kindersley would like to thank the Ramayani Memorial Yoga Institute, Pune for their permission to use photographs of B.K.S. Iyengar from their archives; Sudha Malik, the yoga consultant for the project; Amit Kharsani for the Sanskrit calligraphy; and R.C. Sharma for indexing. The publishers would also like to thank Clare Sheddon and Salima Hirani for their help and advice during the early stages of the project; and Abhijeet Mukherjee for production support.

PICTURE CREDITS

Dorling Kindersley would like to thank the following for their kind permission to reproduce their photographs: National Museum, New Delhi p10, p21 bl, p25 t, p33 t, & b, p35 b, p37; American Institute of Indian Studies, New Delhi p11 tl, p12, p24, p28 t, p39; Max Alexander p22; Akhil Bakshi p13 b, p36; Subhash Bhargava p31; Joe Cornish p29; Andy Crawford p11 tr & b; Antonia Deutch p19 b; Ashok Dilwali p8 , p161; Ashim Ghosh p40; Steve Gorton p11 tr; Alistair Hughes p26; Madan Mohan Jain p13 t (2 photographs superimposed), p34 t; Subir Kumedan p384; Ashok Nath p21; Stephen Parker p6; Janet Peckam p15; Kim Sayer p158; Hashmat Singh p154; Arvind Teki p157; Pankaj Usrani p28 b; Amar Talwar p236; Colin Walton p159 tc. DK Copyright pages (shot by Harminder Singh) 48-49, 56-59, 76-79, 177 b, 178, 182, 183 t, 184-185, 186 tr, 191-195, 199-203, 216-218, 219 t, 222-223, 226-227

Every effort has been made to trace the copyright holders of photographs. The publisher apologizes for any omissions and will amend further editions.

KEY: t=top; r=right; l=left; c=centre; b=bottom

Useful Addresses

B.K.S. Iyengar website: **www.bksiyengar.com**

UNITED KINGDOM & EUROPE

Iyengar Yoga Institute Maida Vale,
223a Randolph Avenue,
Maida Vale,
London W9 1NL

Iyengar Yoga Vidyasthana/ Centre de Yoga Iyengar de Paris,
35 ave.Victor Hugo, Paris 75116, France

Association Francaise de Yoga Iyengar
141, avenue Malakoff, Paris 75016, France

Centre de Yoga Iyengar de Rouen
6, rue Saint Denis, 76000, Rouen, France

Italy Scuola Di Yoga
Via Delle Ruote 49, Firenze 50129, Italy

Centro Iyengar Yoga
18 Via San Gervasio, Firenze 50131, Italy

**Yoga United, Renate Ockel,
Hermann Traitteur**
60 Ansbacher Str., Berlin 10118, Germany

Iyengar Yoga Institute of Amsterdam,
138 Nieuwe Achtergracht, 1018 WV Amsterdam, Netherlands

The Iyengar Yoga Studio,
ul.Przyjaciol Zolnierza, 88/10 71-670, Szczecin, Poland

Centre Espanola de Yoga Iyengar,
Carrera de San Jeronimo 16-5 izda, Madrid 28014, Spain

Institute of Iyengar Yoga and Physiotherapy
Fysikgrand 23 Box 7071 907 03 Umea, Sweden

CANADA

Yoga Centre Toronto
2428 Yonge Street, Toronto, Ontario, Canada M4P 2H4

Centre de Yoga Iyengar de Montréal
919 avenue du Mont-Royal est, Montréal, Québec, Canada H2J 1X3

BKS Iyengar Yoga Association
P.O. Box 48253 Bentall Centre, Vancouver, British Columbia, Canada V7X 1A1

Iyengar Yoga Ottawa Gatineau
784 Bronson Avenue, Ottawa, Ontario, Canada K1S 4G4

USA

Iyengar Yoga Institute of Greater New York,
150 W. 22nd Street, NY 10011, USA

Iyengar Yoga Institute of Los Angeles,
8233 West 3rd Street, LA, CA 90048, USA

Iyengar Yoga Institute of San Francisco,
2404 27th Ave, SF, CA 94116, USA

AUSTRALIA

BKS Iyengar Association of Australia Inc.
P.O Box 159, Mosman
NSW 2088
Tel: 1800 677 037

Yoga Synergy
PO Box 9, Waverley,
NSW 2024
Tel: (02) 9389 7399
www.yogasynergy.com.au

Australian School of Yoga
117 Oxford Street,Bondi Junction,
NSW 2022
Tel: (02) 9389 4694